101 BEST EXERCISES

By Jon Lipsey

Photography **Darren Russell, Glen Burrows**
Models **Donald Akim, Adrian James and Matt Morgan@WAthletic**
Design **Ian Jackson**
Associate Editor **Chris Miller**

With thanks to the Twenty Five Club (the25club.com)

MAG**BOOK**

Publishing Director **Richard Downey**
Deputy Managing Director **James Burnay**
Digital Production Manager **Nicky Baker**
Bookazine Manager **Dharmesh Mistry**
Production Director **Robin Ryan**
Managing Director of Advertising
Julian Lloyd-Evans
Newstrade Director **Martin Belson**
Chief Operating Officer **Brett Reynolds**
Group Finance Director **Ian Leggett**
Chief Executive **James Tye**
Chairman **Felix Dennis**

reflex®

INSTANT WHEY DELUXE

A NEW VARIANT OF INSTANT WHEY WITH AN UNBEATEN TASTE

By taking Instant Whey and increasing the flavor experience and intensity by using the finest ingredients available such as freeze dried strawberry and the richest, darkest cocoa, we're confident that we have created the best tasting whey protein in its class.

FLAVOUR & PERFORMANCE

Instant Whey Deluxe combines an unbeaten taste with a competitive protein level. By using specially selected protein that is rich in peptides and amino acids which are more readily absorbed in the body compared to bonded proteins, an almost instantaneous hit of muscle building amino acids is provided.

It also contains glutamine which has been studied for its unique contribution to protein synthesis, its ability to help prevent muscle tissue breakdown as well as supporting the immune system and assisting cell hydration and volume.

WITH HEALTH FOCUSED INGREDIENTS

Not only does Instant Whey Deluxe combine an unbeaten taste with a competitive protein level, but it also contains health focused ingredients with the inclusion of Digezyme enzymes and Lactospore probiotics. Digezyme enzymes have been shown to enhance protein digestion, whilst Lactospore probiotics, similar to those found in certain yoghurts, provide for a healthier gut.

Instant Whey Deluxe is naturally rich in cysteine which helps promote the body's natural production of Glutathione which is a master antioxidant.

Manufactured by Reflex in one of our three bespoke manufacturing units.

PERFORMANCE & HEALTH WITHIN

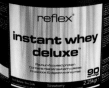
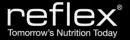

the best sportsmen

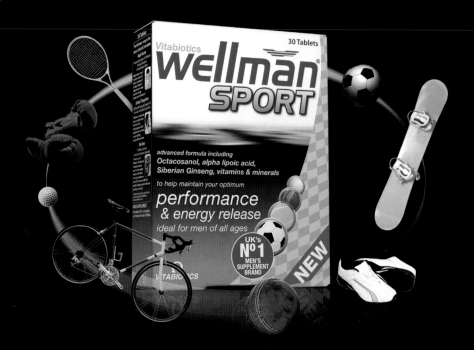

NEW

Vitabiotics
wellman®
SPORT

30 Tablets

advanced formula including
Octacosanol, alpha lipoic acid,
Siberian Ginseng, vitamins & minerals

to help maintain your optimum
performance
& energy release
ideal for men of all ages

UK's
Nº1
MEN'S
SUPPLEMENT
BRAND

NEW

use the best equipment

Wellman® Sport is designed to help support the most important piece of sporting equipment there is – you. Its comprehensive formula safeguards your nutritional requirement to help sustain the body whilst training. The advanced one-a-day tablet replaces your usual multivitamin and includes natural plant isolate Octacosanol, Alpha Lipoic Acid for advanced antioxidant protection and B-complex vitamins to help support energy release. For further information, visit Wellman.co.uk.

Wellman® Sport is new from Wellman®, the UK's leading supplement range for men.

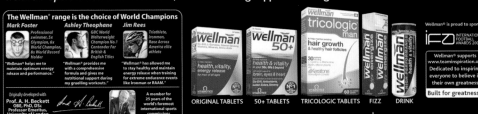

The Wellman® range is the choice of World Champions

Mark Foster
Professional swimmer, 5x Olympian, 6x World Champion, 8x World Record Holder

"Wellman® helps me to maintain optimum energy release and performance."

Ashley Theophane
GBC World Welterweight Champion No.1 Contender For British & English Titles

"Wellman® provides me with a comprehensive formula and gives me nutritional support during my gruelling workouts."

Jim Rees
Triathlete, Ironman, Race Across America elite athlete

"Wellman® has allowed me to stay healthy and maintain energy release when training for extreme endurance events like Ironman or RAAM."

Originally developed with
Prof. A. H. Beckett
OBE, PhD, DSc
Professor Emeritus,
University of London

A member for 25 years of the world's foremost international sports commissions

ORIGINAL TABLETS   **50+ TABLETS**   **TRICOLOGIC TABLETS**   **FIZZ**   **DRINK**

Wellman® is proud to sponsor

iFD INTERNATIONAL FOOTBALL AWARDS 2009

Wellman® supports
www.teaminspiration.org
Dedicated to inspiring everyone to believe in their own greatness
Built for greatness™

Foreword

I f you always do the same exercises every time you train, you'll never get the body you want. To develop a lean, muscular physique you need to vary your workouts so that your body can respond positively to the new stimulus. Now that you have over 100 of the most effective moves at your disposal, complete with detailed form guides, you'll never be short of fresh exercises to use in your routines.

Tailoring workouts to suit your goals

The book is split up into body part sections so if you want to concentrate on a specific goal, such as adding size to your arms, you have an arsenal of the best moves. We've also included a comprehensive guide to creating your own workouts (p8-15), so you can put the moves together for maximum effect.

CONTENTS

8-15
Creating workouts

16-40
Chest and triceps

42-68
Back and biceps

70-96
Abs and core

98-117
Legs

118-129
Shoulders

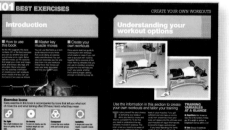

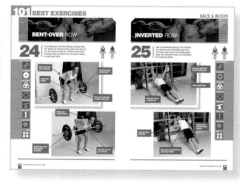

Introduction

■ How to use this book

As the title suggests, this book contains 101 of the best exercises you can do, whether you work out at home or in a gym. We've split the moves up into sections that target your chest and triceps, back and biceps, abs, legs and shoulders. We've also given you the essential information on creating your own workouts, which means that you can use this book in two ways as follows.

■ Master key muscle moves

You can use this book as a form guide resource so you know that you're doing an exercise safely and effectively. You can also pick exercises you like and drop them into your workouts. Doing these new moves will keep your body stimulated and help you build muscle.

■ Create your own workouts

Once you've read our guide to creating your own workouts, which starts on page 9, you can start to put your own routines together. We've covered all the major training variables that you can use to construct a training programme that will help you reach your goals, whether that's getting bigger, getting stronger or shedding body fat.

Exercise icons

Every exercise in this book is accompanied by icons that tell you what sort of move it is and what training effect it'll have. Here's what they mean

Go light
Use a light resistance and focus on getting the form right.

Go heavy
To pack on muscle, use the heaviest weight you can handle safely.

Compound
A move that uses multiple joints and muscle groups.

Isolation
A single-joint move that targets a specific muscle group.

Stabiliser
A move that requires you to hold your body steady.

Explosive
These moves should be done quickly and powerfully.

Core
Exercises that train the muscles around your midriff.

Form alert
Pay particular attention to correct form to avoid injuries to muscles.

Understanding your workout options

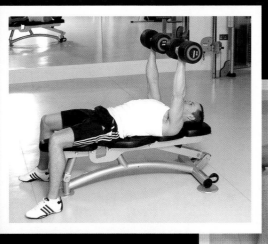
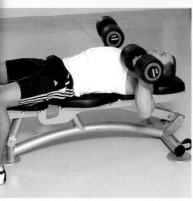

Use the information in this section to create your own workouts and tailor your training

o give yourself the best chance of achieving your workout aims, you need to create and stick to a programme. To do that you need to understand the key variables involved in exercise. The main ones you need to be aware of, and the ones addressed here, are reps, sets, rest, tempo and frequency.

How muscles grow
A basic understanding of what happens to your muscles when you exercise will help you use the training variables effectively. Performing resistance exercises creates tiny tears in your muscles. If you get sufficient rest and take on amino acids from protein-rich food your body will respond to this stimulus and your muscles will repair themselves to become bigger and stronger.

If you keep repeating the same workout, though, your body will adapt to the stimulus and your progress will stall. That's why you need a broad range of exercises, such as the 101 in this book, at your disposal. Using the key training variables will further increase your workout options and help you get the body you've always wanted.

TRAINING VARIABLES AT A GLANCE

■ **Repetitions** Also known as reps, this is the number of times you lift a weight or perform a bodyweight exercise within a set.

■ **Sets** Groups of repetitions performed back to back.

■ **Rest** The inactive time you take between sets and exercises.

■ **Tempo** The speed at which reps are performed.

■ **Frequency** This refers to how often you perform a workout.

Repetitions

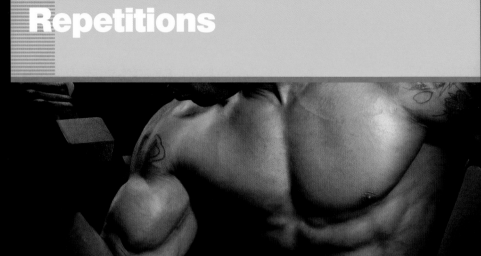

The number of repetitions you perform will affect your results. Here's how to use different rep ranges to meet your goals

You might think that more reps equals more muscle, but that's not the case. The number of repetitions you perform each set will have a big impact on whether the primary effect of your workout is developing muscle strength, size or endurance. Low reps in the one-to-six range are best for building strength; between seven and 12 reps is best for adding muscle mass; and 13 or more reps will develop muscle endurance.

These are, however, broad guides and are on a spectrum rather than self-contained blocks. Performing three or six repetitions of an exercise, for example, will build strength but doing six repetitions will have more of a size development effect than performing three, because it's closer to the size gain range of the spectrum.

Fail to succeed

In each case, to get the desired effect, you should aim to reach failure (when you can't complete another rep without compromising form) at your target rep count on the final set of the exercise. If you complete your reps and feel that you could perform more, you're not using a heavy enough weight.

Reps at a glance

Effect	Reps
Strength	1-6
Muscle mass	7-12
Endurance	13+

It's also important to remember that these rep ranges are general guides. Not everyone responds to resistance training in exactly the same way and even different muscles in the body can respond differently, depending on their function. For example, slow-twitch muscle fibres (the smaller muscle fibres involved in long-distance endurance efforts) will generally experience strength gains at a higher rep range than fast-twitch muscle fibres (the larger muscle fibres involved in short, explosive movements).

Your level of training experience will also play a part in your results. Generally, people new to weight training will develop strength into a slightly higher rep range than more experienced exercisers.

Sets

Pick the right number to fatigue your muscles and get stronger

How many sets you perform is directly related to how many reps you do. Generally, the more sets you do, the fewer reps you should perform and vice versa.

Doing three sets of ten to 12 reps is a standard formula that will allow you to lift enough weight to challenge your muscles and also fatigue them in a time that will maximise your training effect. If you tried to do six sets of ten to 12 reps it would be almost impossible to pick a weight that would give you a decent training effect and allow you to complete all the reps.

Even if you could complete them, your workouts would take too long. Studies show that the most effective workout length for building strength and muscle is 45 minutes. After that your training efforts can be counterproductive, because testosterone levels drop and stress hormone levels rise. That also means that if you include a high number of exercises in your workout you may need to reduce the sets per exercise you perform.

Experience matters

If you're new to training, you may consider doing one or two sets of each exercise to get your muscles used to performing the movements. As you improve, you can increase the total number of sets you complete. Experienced lifters often get better strength and hypertrophy (muscle growth) results by doing higher numbers of sets with lower numbers of reps.

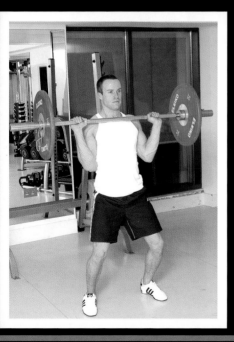
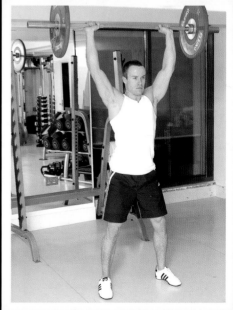

Tempo

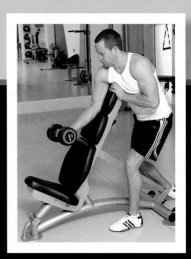

Make sure you're lifting at the most effective speed

The speed at which you perform your exercises will contribute to their training effect. Don't bash out your reps as fast as you can because you're likely to use momentum, rather than your own strength, to shift the weight. You're also likely to compromise your form, which could lead to injury, and you won't be putting your muscles under tension for the optimum amount of time.

To maximise strength and size improvements, research suggests your muscles should be under tension for between 40 and 70 seconds per set, provided you're not using low rep ranges. This will cause you to use anaerobic energy, which produces lactate and prompts the release of testosterone and growth hormones.

You also need to pay attention to the tempo you use to complete each part of a lift. To make sure your muscles are under tension for long enough, take one second to lift the weight, pause, then take two to three seconds to lower. The reason you take longer to lower is that size gains are best made during the eccentric (lowering) phase of the lift.

Taking your time will help you recruit stabilising muscles, which protect your joints and support the bigger muscles when you attempt heavy lifts. It also takes momentum out of the exercises.

Lifting and lowering

Some exercises, such as the clean and press, have to be performed at speed because they require explosive movements to lift a weight that's heavy enough to have a training benefit. You also generally re-set after each lift, rather than lowering slowly under control. As with sets and reps, it's important to vary the tempo, so don't use the same speed for every exercise and every workout.

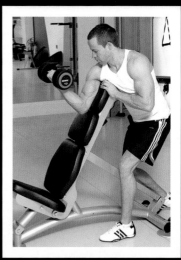

Workout tips

■ Warm up before a workout
Raise your body temperature to prepare for exercise. Run or cycle for five minutes, then do bodyweight exercises such as press-ups or lunges.

■ ...and warm down afterwards
Stretching at the end of your session will help flush out the lactic acid from your muscles and prevent post-exercise soreness and stiffness.

■ Engage your core
Before you start any lift you should engage your core muscles by tensing your midsection. This will keep you stable and protect your back form injury.

■ Eat after exercise
Aim to eat a snack containing fast-acting carbs within 40 minutes of finishing your workout. The carbs will top up your energy stores and the protein will help build muscle.

Rest

Use recovery periods to make your workout effective

The rest you take between sets and exercises determines whether or not you're able to complete the next section of your workout. As a rule, sets with few reps will require the most rest. This is because they train the nervous system and fast-twitch muscle fibres, which fatigue easily and take longer to recover. You may need to rest for up to five minutes when you perform low reps of an explosive move with heavy weights. As you increase the number of reps you train more slow-twitch muscle fibres, which are harder to fatigue.

Vary your rests

Different exercises also require different rest times. Big compound moves such as squats and deadlifts require longer rests of about two minutes than single joint isolation moves, which may only require 30 seconds' rest between exercises.

If you are new to weight training you may need to take longer rests than more experienced lifters, who have a higher tolerance to the lactate produced during lifts. How much you weigh can also affect your rest times, with heavier lifters needing longer to recover between sets.

Essentially, your rest periods are effective when you can reach positive failure on the last rep of the set. This means that you are unable to lift the weight with perfect form but are able to lower it under control. If you don't reach that point by the end of your set, make sure that you are sticking to your rest periods.

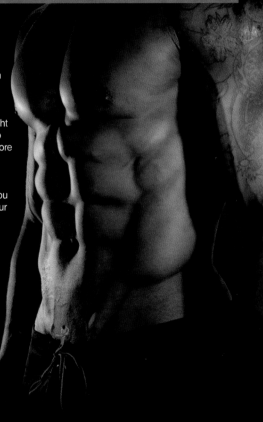

■ Don't ignore pain
The phrase 'no pain no gain' is nonsense. You do need to push yourself and put effort into your workouts but if you feel pain, stop.

■ Get your form right
Follow the form guides that annotate each exercise and you'll reduce your chances of getting injured. Ignore them and you'll end up on the treatment table.

■ Go big to get bigger
Big multi-muscle exercises such as squats and deadlifts are the most effective for building muscle. They place a high demand on your body and they burn more calories.

■ See your GP
If you're new to exercise or you have any concerns about the state of your health, go for a check-up with your GP.

Frequency

How many workouts should you do each week? Here's what you need to know

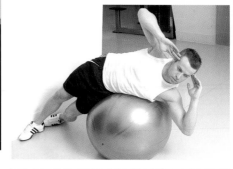

For most people, the biggest barrier to fitness is not having enough time to work out. But the good news is that you don't need to train seven days a week to see great results. Doing three workouts a week should be sufficient to achieve your workout goals.

Exactly how many sessions you do depends on a number of factors. One thing that should influence training frequency is what sort of workouts you're doing. A hard fully-body session may mean that you need to leave at least 48 hours between sessions in order for your muscles to recover. If you're focusing on a particular body part each workout, you may be able to train the following day if you work on a different body part.

Less is more

One common mistake is to think that the more workouts you do, the stronger and more muscular you'll become. In fact it's while you're resting, rather than while you're working out, that your muscles get bigger and stronger. If you stress your muscles before they've had a chance to repair themselves this may cause overtraining, where you lose strength and muscle mass and feel lethargic.

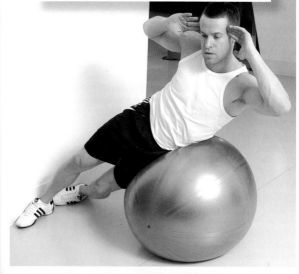

Some muscle groups take longer to recover than others. Larger muscle groups, particularly those with a comparatively higher percentage of fast-twitch muscle fibres, such as the hamstrings, may take longer to recover than smaller muscle groups such as the calves.

Doing big compound lifts such as deadlifts also places more of a stress on your nervous system than smaller lifts, such as biceps curls, so you'll need longer to recover. You should also take longer to recover from intense sessions, where you do low reps of heavy weights, than you do from endurance and stability sessions, where you do high reps of light weights.

Selecting and ordering exercises

Here's how to structure your workouts for maximum effect

The following guidelines will help you to structure your workouts to maximise muscle growth and strength gains and to minimise injury risk.

Do difficult moves first and easier moves last
Perform large muscle group moves, such as squats and deadlifts, at the beginning of your workout to make sure you keep perfect form and your core is strong enough to stabilise your body. Easier moves, such as biceps curls, should be done later in the workout.

Do big explosive moves early in your workout
Explosive exercises such as the hang clean are very demanding so they need to be performed when you are relatively fresh. Do these moves earlier in your workout than simpler moves such as triceps extensions.

Keep your workouts balanced
Unless you are specifically doing an unbalanced workout (one made up exclusively of pushing movements, for example), it's advisable to try to keep your workouts balanced. So

for every pushing exercise you do, you should do a pulling one.

Save core moves until last
If you do core moves early on in your workout you'll fatigue the muscles. When you then come to do big dynamic lifts, such as lunges, that call on your core to stabilise your movement, they may not be able to provide adequate support, which can increase your injury risk.

SAMPLE WORKOUTS

■ All-body workout

Exercise	Sets	Reps	Page
Pull-up	3	8	52
Squat	3	10	101
Bench press	3	10	18
Lunge	2	10 each side	110
Shoulder press	3	10	120
Dumb-bell biceps curl	2	10 each side	62
Gym ball crunch	3	12	77
Plank	3	30-60 seconds	76

■ Body focus workout (shoulders)

Exercise	Sets	Reps	Page
Internal cable row	2	15 each side	128
External cable row	2	15 each side	129
Clean and press	3	8	59
Push press	3	10	121
Cuban press	3	12	127
Lateral raise	3	12	125

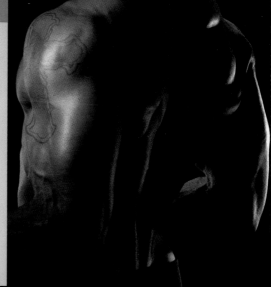

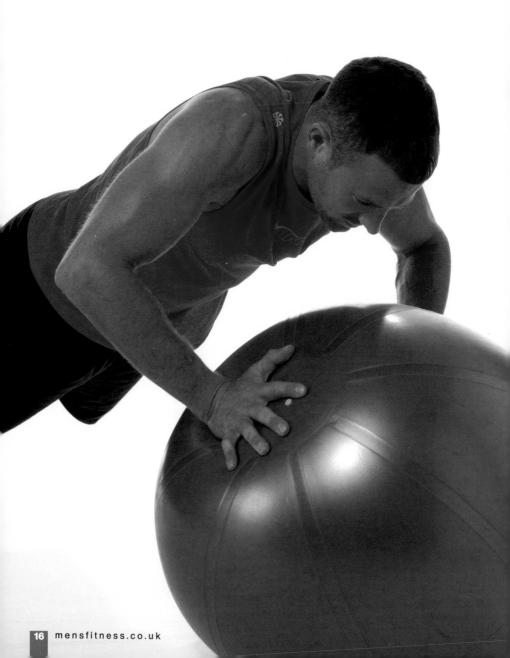

Chest & triceps

These muscle groups have been put together because they are frequently used in the same moves. Any press-up variation, for example, as well as bench presses, are powered by both your chest and triceps.

Chest

The main job of the chest muscles – the pectorals or 'pecs' – is to push your arms in front of you, although they are also used when bringing your arms down in front of you. There are two main muscles in this group.

The pectoralis major is a large muscle that attaches to your collarbone, breastbone and ribs. Although it is a single muscle, most experienced weight trainers divide the chest into three portions: upper, middle and lower. Any chest exercise will work the entire muscle, but by varying the angle of attack – by doing incline or decline bench presses, for example – it is possible to target the upper or lower portions of the chest.

The pectoralis minor is a thin triangular muscle in the upper part of the chest near the shoulder and below the pectoralis major. Its function is to bring the shoulder forward, an important part of generating strength in big chest moves such as bench presses.

Triceps

The biceps may get most of the training attention but the triceps makes up two-thirds of your upper arm muscle mass. As its the name suggests, it's made up of three 'heads' – lateral, long and medial. The lateral and medial heads of the triceps are involved in straightening your arm, while the long head is engaged when you draw your arms down in front of you.

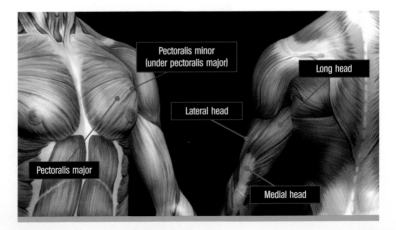

Pectoralis minor
(under pectoralis major)

Long head

Lateral head

Pectoralis major

Medial head

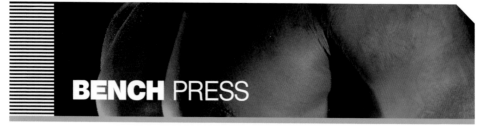

BENCH PRESS

01

This is *the* classic chest-building move and a standard test of upper-body strength. It is also a great all-over mass-builder because it requires a large number of muscle fibres to perform, which triggers the body's natural growth hormone response.

LIGHT WEIGHTS

GO HEAVY

COMPOUND

ISOLATION

STABILISER

FORM ALERT

EXPLOSIVE

CORE

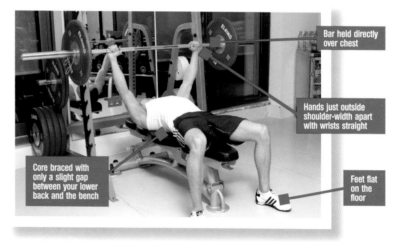

Bar held directly over chest

Hands just outside shoulder-width apart with wrists straight

Core braced with only a slight gap between your lower back and the bench

Feet flat on the floor

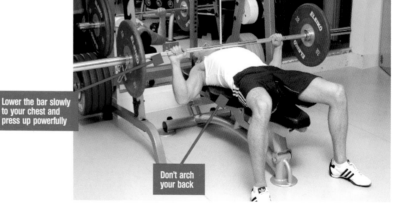

Lower the bar slowly to your chest and press up powerfully

Don't arch your back

PRESS-UP

02

The equivalent of a bodyweight bench press. Because you control your own weight, the press-up has more real-world usefulness than the bench press but is less effective at building mass because it is hard to vary the resistance. Use it to build endurance and strengthen shoulder stabilisers.

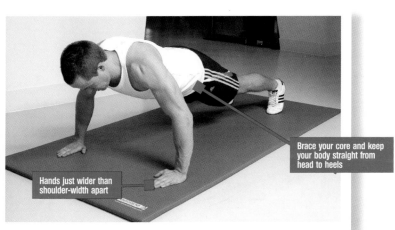

Hands just wider than shoulder-width apart

Brace your core and keep your body straight from head to heels

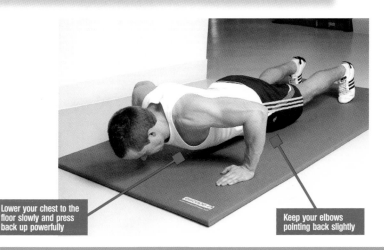

Lower your chest to the floor slowly and press back up powerfully

Keep your elbows pointing back slightly

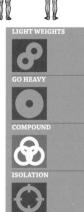

LIGHT WEIGHTS

GO HEAVY

COMPOUND

ISOLATION

STABILISER

FORM ALERT

EXPLOSIVE

CORE

CABLE CROSSOVER

03

By using a cable machine, you keep the tension on your muscles constant throughout the move. Your midriff will also get a workout keeping your torso stable against the cables' resistance.

LIGHT WEIGHTS

GO HEAVY

COMPOUND

ISOLATION

STABILISER

FORM ALERT

EXPLOSIVE

CORE

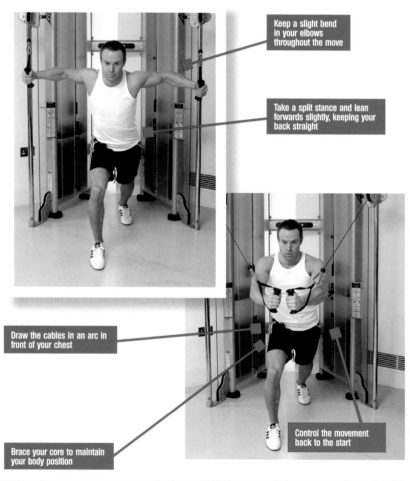

Keep a slight bend in your elbows throughout the move

Take a split stance and lean forwards slightly, keeping your back straight

Draw the cables in an arc in front of your chest

Brace your core to maintain your body position

Control the movement back to the start

DUMB-BELL PULLOVER

04

Target your chest from a new angle by pulling the weight over your head. This targets the lower portion of your pectorals and also works your lats – the 'wings' down the sides of your back.

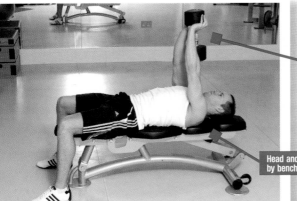

Grasp a dumb-bell in both hands above your head

Head and shoulders supported by bench, and feet on the floor

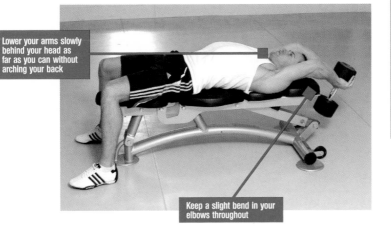

Lower your arms slowly behind your head as far as you can without arching your back

Keep a slight bend in your elbows throughout

LIGHT WEIGHTS

GO HEAVY

COMPOUND

ISOLATION

STABILISER

FORM ALERT

EXPLOSIVE

CORE

DUMB-BELL
BENCH PRESS

05

Dumb-bells have certain advantages over the barbell. You get a more natural range of motion, which means less stress on delicate shoulder joints, and each arm works independently so you get more even growth. The downside is that you won't be able to shift as much weight as with a barbell.

LIGHT WEIGHTS

GO HEAVY

COMPOUND

ISOLATION

STABILISER

FORM ALERT

EXPLOSIVE

CORE

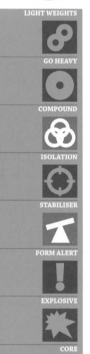

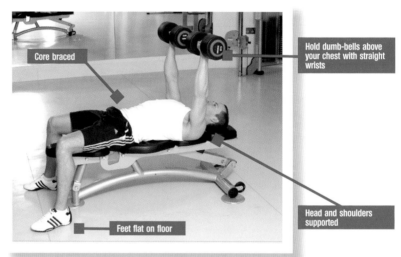

Core braced

Hold dumb-bells above your chest with straight wrists

Head and shoulders supported

Feet flat on floor

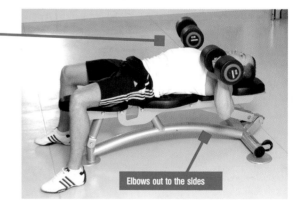

Lower the weights slowly to chest level and then press back up powerfully

Elbows out to the sides

PASSING MEDICINE BALL
PRESS-UP

06

For greater functional strength and improved sporting performance, this exercise forces your muscles cope with awkward angles, unstable surfaces and coordinated movements. Perform it quickly without compromising good form.

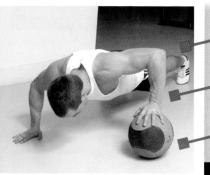

Feet apart for stability

Maintain a straight body from head to heels

Place one hand on a medicine ball

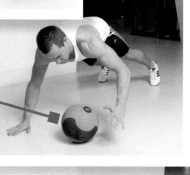

Perform a press-up and, as you rise up, roll the ball over to the other hand

Roll the ball back and forth with each press-up

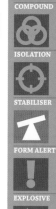

LIGHT WEIGHTS

GO HEAVY

COMPOUND

ISOLATION

STABILISER

FORM ALERT

EXPLOSIVE

CORE

INCLINE
BENCH PRESS

07 Set the bench at an angle to shift the emphasis to the upper portion of your pectorals.

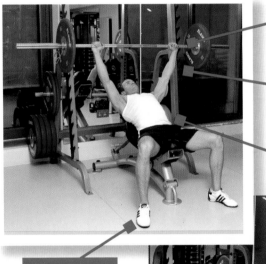

Hold the bar directly above your chest

Hands just wider than shoulder-width apart

Set the bench at a 30°-45° angle

Feet flat on the floor

Lower the bar slowly to your chest and press back up powerfully

Keep your core braced throughout and don't arch your back

DUMB-BELL FLYE

08

This exercise takes your triceps out of the equation, placing most of the impact on your chest muscles. The movement puts a fair amount of stress on your shoulders, so start with a light weight and build up slowly.

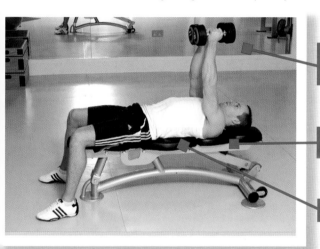

Hold dumb-bells above your chest with palms facing inwards

Head and shoulders supported by bench

Brace your core

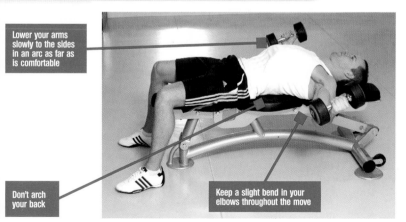

Lower your arms slowly to the sides in an arc as far as is comfortable

Don't arch your back

Keep a slight bend in your elbows throughout the move

LIGHT WEIGHTS

GO HEAVY

COMPOUND

ISOLATION

STABILISER

FORM ALERT

EXPLOSIVE

CORE

DECLINE BENCH PRESS

09

Adjust your bench so your head is pointing down and you'll work the lower part of your chest muscles.

LIGHT WEIGHTS

GO HEAVY

COMPOUND

ISOLATION

STABILISER

FORM ALERT

EXPLOSIVE

CORE

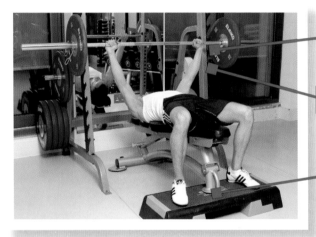

Hold the bar directly above your chest

Hands just wider than shoulder-width apart

If you don't have a special decline bench, raise the end of a flat bench on a low platform

Lower the bar slowly to your chest and press back up powerfully

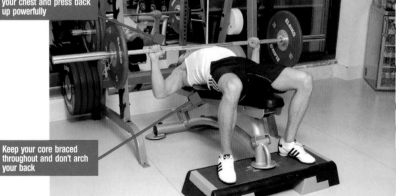

Keep your core braced throughout and don't arch your back

GYM BALL
PRESS-UP

10

Keeping the ball steady while you lower and raise your body requires excellent muscle control. Use this move to stimulate under-used muscles that will, at a later date, help to improve your bench press.

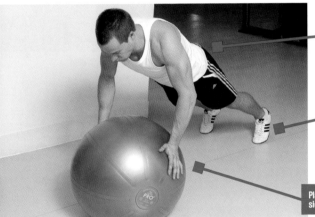

Body straight from head to heels

Feet apart for stability

Place one hand on each side of the ball

LIGHT WEIGHTS

GO HEAVY

COMPOUND

ISOLATION

STABILISER

FORM ALERT

EXPLOSIVE

CORE

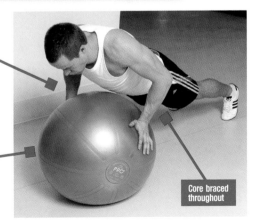

Lower your chest slowly to the ball and press back up

Try to control the wobble of the ball as you move

Core braced throughout

T PRESS-UP

11

Add a dynamic rotational element to the plain old press-up to turn it into a fat-torching power move. The trick is to make the exercise fast and fluid, using your core muscles to control the movement.

LIGHT WEIGHTS

GO HEAVY

COMPOUND

ISOLATION

STABILISER

FORM ALERT

EXPLOSIVE

CORE

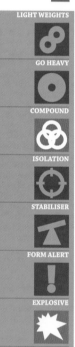

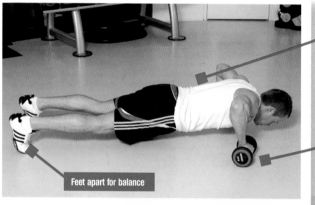

Body straight from head to heels

Hold light dumb-bells with straight wrists

Feet apart for balance

Press up and rotate your body to the side, lifting your arm

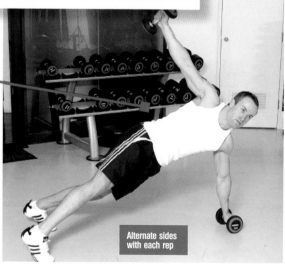

Alternate sides with each rep

BENCH DIP

12

A simple, effective way to work your triceps, the bench dip is a good starting point before you move on to parallel bar dips (see p34). The position it places your shoulders in can put strain on your shoulder joint, so take care if you have existing shoulder problems and build up your range of motion slowly.

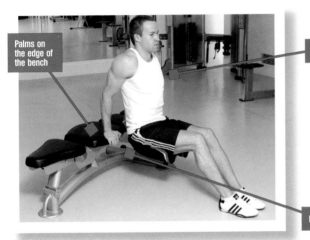

Palms on the edge of the bench

Keep your torso upright

Back close to the bench

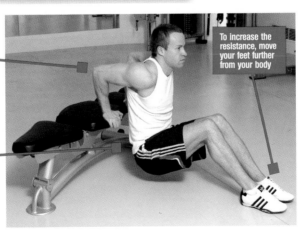

Keep your elbows pointing back

To increase the resistance, move your feet further from your body

Lower your body as far as is comfortable

LIGHT WEIGHTS

GO HEAVY

COMPOUND

ISOLATION

STABILISER

FORM ALERT

EXPLOSIVE

CORE

CLOSE-GRIP
BENCH PRESS

13

By moving your hands closer together on the bar, you transfer the emphasis from your chest to your triceps. The close grip also makes the bar more difficult to control, so use a lighter weight than you would on a conventional bench press until you are confident of increasing it.

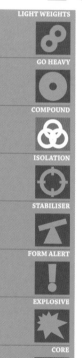

LIGHT WEIGHTS

GO HEAVY

COMPOUND

ISOLATION

STABILISER

FORM ALERT

EXPLOSIVE

CORE

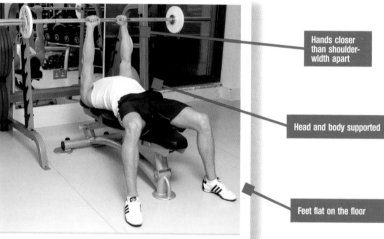

Hands closer than shoulder-width apart

Head and body supported

Feet flat on the floor

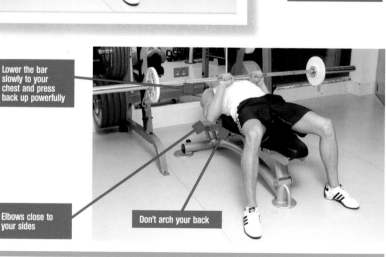

Lower the bar slowly to your chest and press back up powerfully

Elbows close to your sides

Don't arch your back

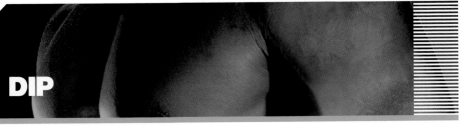

DIP

14

The dip should be utilised by anyone looking to add solid mass to their triceps. Once you can manage ten to 15 dips with perfect form, you can increase the resistance by hanging weight plates from a belt. Be careful if you have shoulder problems, however, because this move can exacerbate them.

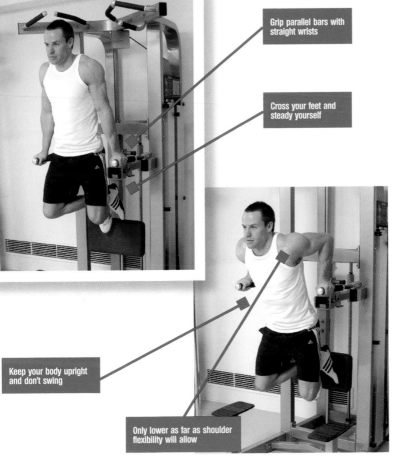

Grip parallel bars with straight wrists

Cross your feet and steady yourself

Keep your body upright and don't swing

Only lower as far as shoulder flexibility will allow

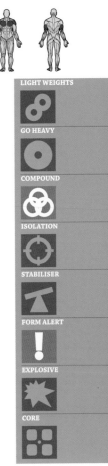

LIGHT WEIGHTS

GO HEAVY

COMPOUND

ISOLATION

STABILISER

FORM ALERT

EXPLOSIVE

CORE

ROPE PRESS-DOWN

15

By turning your wrists out at the bottom of the move you get an intense contraction on the triceps. You may find you have to use lighter weights as a result.

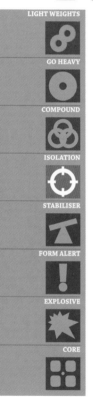

LIGHT WEIGHTS

GO HEAVY

COMPOUND

ISOLATION

STABILISER

FORM ALERT

EXPLOSIVE

CORE

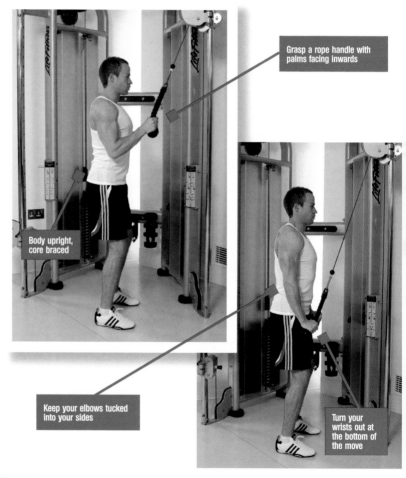

Grasp a rope handle with palms facing inwards

Body upright, core braced

Keep your elbows tucked into your sides

Turn your wrists out at the bottom of the move

EZ-BAR OVERHEAD
TRICEPS EXTENSION

16

Stand up, load up and target your triceps with a heavyweight move.

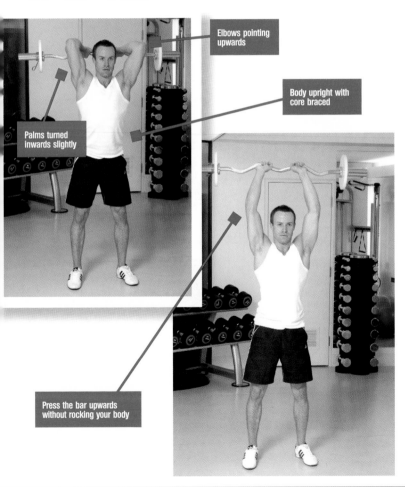

Elbows pointing upwards

Body upright with core braced

Palms turned inwards slightly

Press the bar upwards without rocking your body

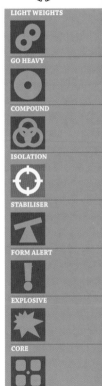

LIGHT WEIGHTS

GO HEAVY

COMPOUND

ISOLATION

STABILISER

FORM ALERT

EXPLOSIVE

CORE

CLAP PRESS-UP

17

A good exercise for show-offs! If you can crank out 12 reps of these, then you can consider yourself officially strong. The explosive nature of the move fires up your fast-twitch muscle fibres – the ones that have the most potential for growth.

LIGHT WEIGHTS

GO HEAVY

COMPOUND

ISOLATION

STABILISER

FORM ALERT

EXPLOSIVE

CORE

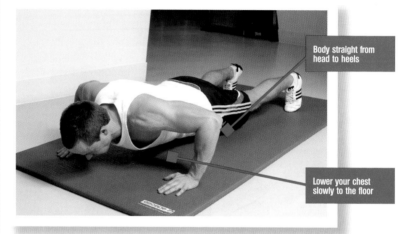

Body straight from head to heels

Lower your chest slowly to the floor

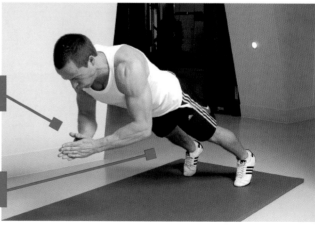

Push up powerfully so that your hands leave the floor – and clap!

Land with bent elbows to absorb the impact

DIAMOND PRESS-UP

18

Placing your hands close together for a press-up puts more pressure on your triceps and less on your chest. Keep the movement slow and controlled to teach your triceps to control your bodyweight.

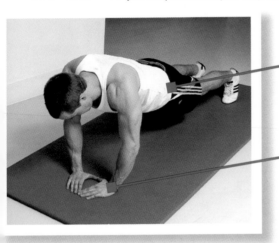

Body straight from head to heels

Touch your thumbs and forefingers together to form a diamond shape

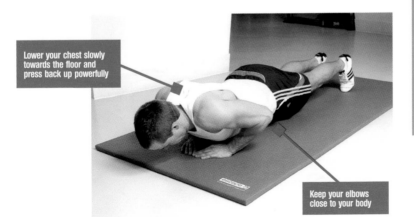

Lower your chest slowly towards the floor and press back up powerfully

Keep your elbows close to your body

LIGHT WEIGHTS

GO HEAVY

COMPOUND

ISOLATION

STABILISER

FORM ALERT

EXPLOSIVE

CORE

MEDICINE BALL
CLOSE-GRIP PRESS-UP

19

The medicine ball introduces a wobbly surface to the press-up, making the stabilising muscles in your shoulders and core work overtime.

LIGHT WEIGHTS

GO HEAVY

COMPOUND

ISOLATION

STABILISER

FORM ALERT

EXPLOSIVE

CORE

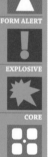

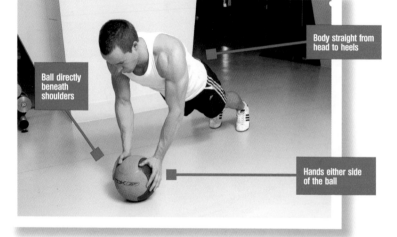

Body straight from head to heels

Ball directly beneath shoulders

Hands either side of the ball

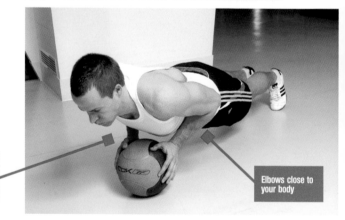

Lower your chest slowly to the ball

Elbows close to your body

CABLE PULLOVER

20

By using a cable instead of a dumb-bell for the pullover, you can keep the resistance on your muscles constant throughout the move, whereas with the dumb-bell the resistance drops off as you raise your arms.

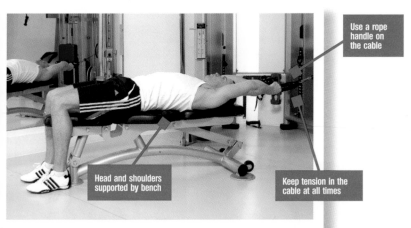

Use a rope handle on the cable

Head and shoulders supported by bench

Keep tension in the cable at all times

LIGHT WEIGHTS

GO HEAVY

COMPOUND

ISOLATION

STABILISER

FORM ALERT

EXPLOSIVE

CORE

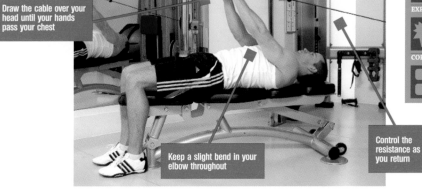

Draw the cable over your head until your hands pass your chest

Keep a slight bend in your elbow throughout

Control the resistance as you return

SEATED ONE-ARM OVERHEAD
TRICEPS EXTENSION

21

The toughest part of this move is just as you begin to raise the weight, which is why it's a good exercise to partner with the dumb-bell kickback (see p33) where the hardest part is when the arm is at full extension.

LIGHT WEIGHTS

GO HEAVY

COMPOUND

ISOLATION

STABILISER

FORM ALERT

EXPLOSIVE

CORE

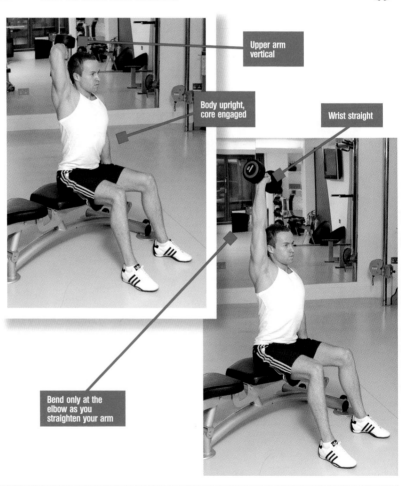

Upper arm vertical

Body upright, core engaged

Wrist straight

Bend only at the elbow as you straighten your arm

NEUTRAL-GRIP
DUMB-BELL PRESS

22

Perform the press with palms facing each other to transfer some of the emphasis away from your chest and onto your triceps. It will also have a different training effect on your shoulders, helping to strengthen your rotator cuff.

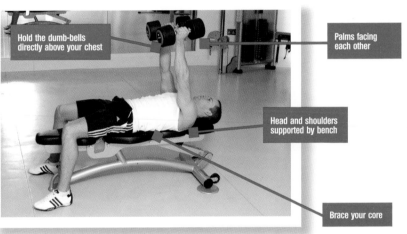

Hold the dumb-bells directly above your chest

Palms facing each other

Head and shoulders supported by bench

Brace your core

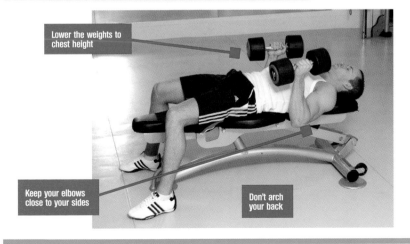

Lower the weights to chest height

Keep your elbows close to your sides

Don't arch your back

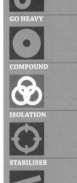

LIGHT WEIGHTS

GO HEAVY

COMPOUND

ISOLATION

STABILISER

FORM ALERT

EXPLOSIVE

CORE

101 BEST EXERCISES

EZ-BAR LYING
TRICEPS EXTENSION

23 The EZ-bar allows you to press heavier weights than you could with dumb-bells, while holding your wrists at an angle that is less stressful than the angle when holding a straight barbell.

LIGHT WEIGHTS

GO HEAVY

COMPOUND

ISOLATION

STABILISER

FORM ALERT

EXPLOSIVE

CORE

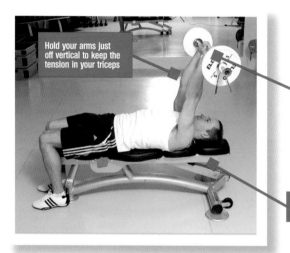

Hold your arms just off vertical to keep the tension in your triceps

Grasp the EZ-bar with your wrists turned in slightly

Head and shoulders supported by the bench

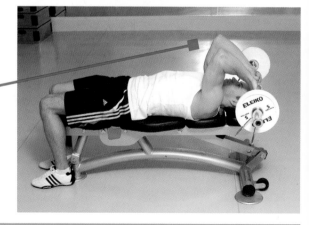

Bend only at the elbows, keeping your upper arms still

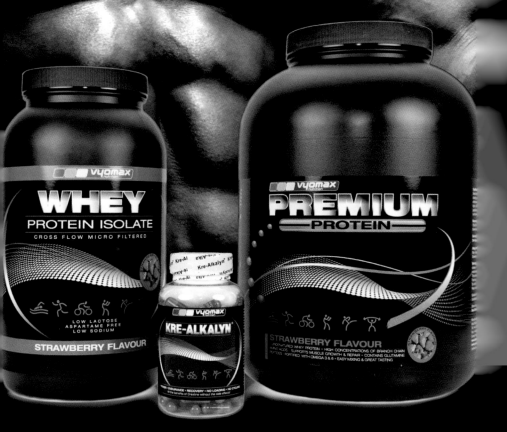

VYOMAX
NUTRITION

FREE SAMPLES
NOW AVAILABLE
QUOTE REF: VYOMAX-1

ORDER ONLINE AT WWW.VYOMAXNUTRITION.COM
TELEPHONE US ON 0161 865 8555 OR EMAIL: SALES@SKSPORTS.CO.UK
AVAILABLE FROM ALL GOOD GYMS, SPORTS NUTRITION AND HEALTH FOOD SHOPS

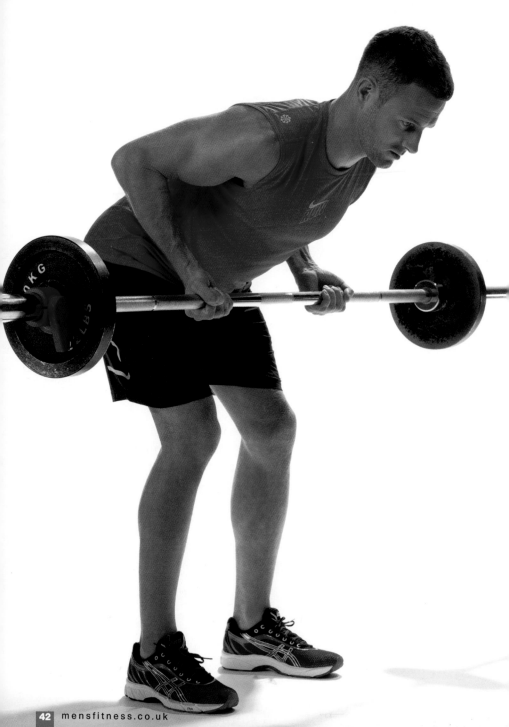

Back & biceps

We've paired these two muscle groups because they're often used together during the same exercise. When you do a reverse-grip bent-over row, for example, both your back and biceps are working hard to move the weight.

Back

Most men would rather train their chest by doing bench presses than spend a session working on their back. But if you neglect the area you'll get bad posture and hunched shoulders as your overdeveloped pecs draw your shoulders forwards. A strong back will help you lift big weights as well as giving you a broad and imposing physique.

At the top of the back are the muscles that control your shoulders.

Your trapezius muscles ('traps') pull your shoulder blades up and together while your rhomboids pull your shoulders back. The latissimus dorsi muscles ('lats') are the large ones down the sides of your back and are responsible for drawing your arms down and back.

Biceps

Getting bigger biceps is a popular workout goal but they're actually a relatively small muscle. The biceps brachii is made up of two parts and is responsible for bending your arm. When your palms are facing down, the muscle that bends your arm is the brachialis. The final muscle in the group is the brachioradialis at the top of your forearm which is responsible for flexing the elbow.

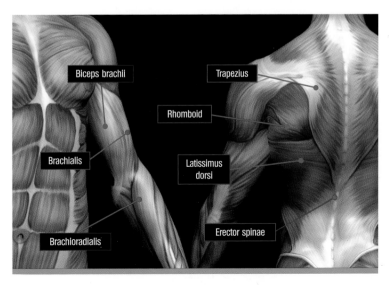

Biceps brachii

Trapezius

Rhomboid

Brachialis

Latissimus dorsi

Brachioradialis

Erector spinae

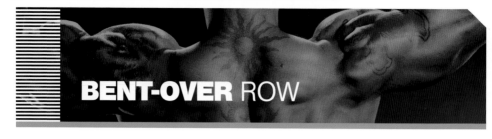

BENT-OVER ROW

24

A powerhouse move for building a strong back. You should be doing as many bent-over rows as you do bench presses to maintain a balanced physique. Ensure perfect form to prevent strains in your lower back.

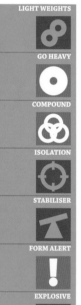

- LIGHT WEIGHTS
- GO HEAVY
- COMPOUND
- ISOLATION
- STABILISER
- FORM ALERT
- EXPLOSIVE
- CORE

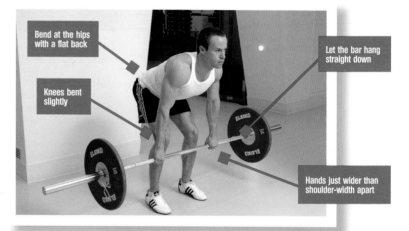

Bend at the hips with a flat back

Knees bent slightly

Let the bar hang straight down

Hands just wider than shoulder-width apart

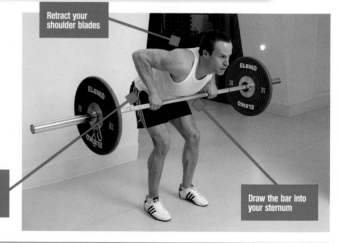

Retract your shoulder blades

Maintain the same body position throughout

Draw the bar into your sternum

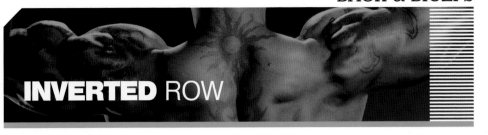

INVERTED ROW

25 Like a backwards press-up, the inverted row requires you to stabilise your core and work against your own bodyweight. Keep the movement slow and controlled for maximum effect.

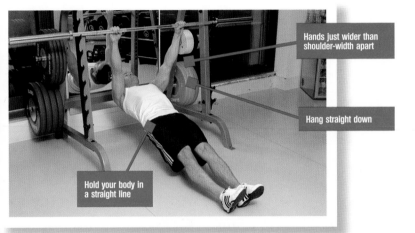

Hands just wider than shoulder-width apart

Hang straight down

Hold your body in a straight line

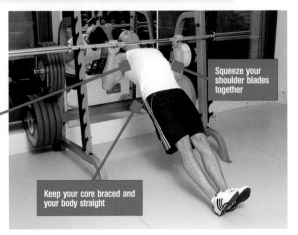

Pull your chest to the bar

Squeeze your shoulder blades together

Keep your core braced and your body straight

LIGHT WEIGHTS

GO HEAVY

COMPOUND

ISOLATION

STABILISER

FORM ALERT

EXPLOSIVE

CORE

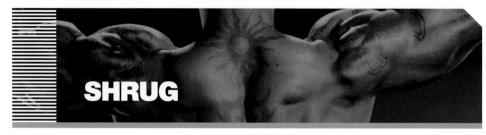

SHRUG

26

The big move for training your upper traps. There's not a lot of movement in this exercise, so you can afford to go as heavy as you dare. Be sure to hold the contraction at the top for a second or two before lowering.

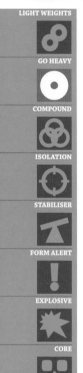

LIGHT WEIGHTS

GO HEAVY

COMPOUND

ISOLATION

STABILISER

FORM ALERT

EXPLOSIVE

CORE

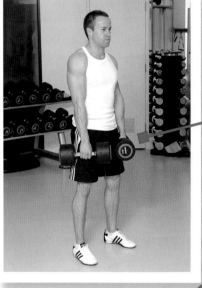

Hold weights on the outside of your thighs (slightly forward)

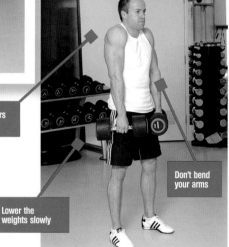

Raise your shoulders towards your ears

Don't bend your arms

Lower the weights slowly

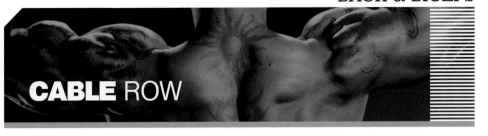

CABLE ROW

27

Another chance to target a large number of muscle fibres in your back and stimulate the body's natural growth hormone response. Avoid the temptation to rock back and forth as you row, because this will transfer the stress to your lower back.

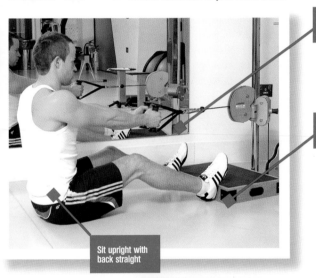

Neutral grip – palms facing each other

Brace your feet with knees bent

Sit upright with back straight

LIGHT WEIGHTS

GO HEAVY

COMPOUND

ISOLATION

STABILISER

FORM ALERT

EXPLOSIVE

CORE

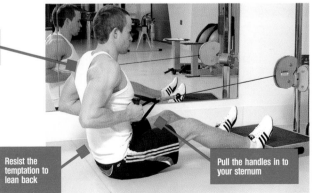

Retract your shoulder blades

Resist the temptation to lean back

Pull the handles in to your sternum

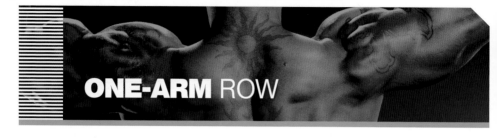

ONE-ARM ROW

28

The unilateral nature of this exercise means that you can iron out any imbalances in your back development brought on by having one arm stronger than the other.

LIGHT WEIGHTS

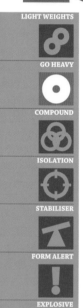

GO HEAVY

COMPOUND

ISOLATION

STABILISER

FORM ALERT

EXPLOSIVE

CORE

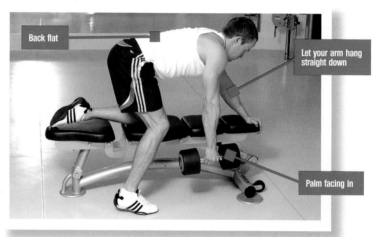

Back flat

Let your arm hang straight down

Palm facing in

Pull the weight in to your side

Lower slowly

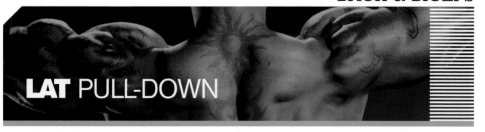

LAT PULL-DOWN

29

This targets your 'wings' – the latissimus dorsi muscles down the sides of your back. If you are aiming to shift heavy weights, you will need a specific lat pull-down machine on which you can jam your knees beneath pads to prevent your body lifting up.

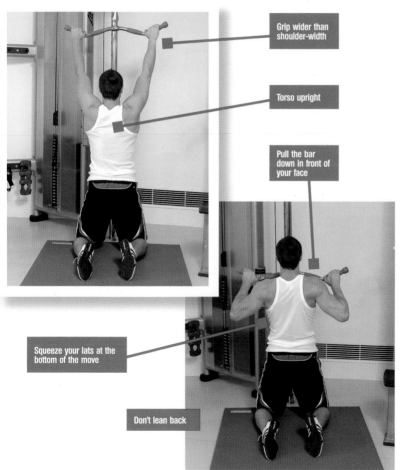

Grip wider than shoulder-width

Torso upright

Pull the bar down in front of your face

Squeeze your lats at the bottom of the move

Don't lean back

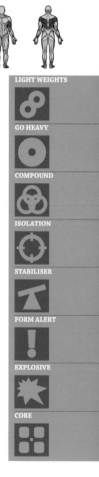

LIGHT WEIGHTS

GO HEAVY

COMPOUND

ISOLATION

STABILISER

FORM ALERT

EXPLOSIVE

CORE

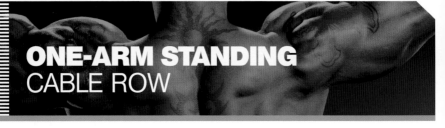

ONE-ARM STANDING
CABLE ROW

30

Using a shoulder-height cable means you target not just the upper part of your back – your trapezius and rhomboids – but your rear shoulders as well. Keep a strong core to prevent your body twisting as you pull.

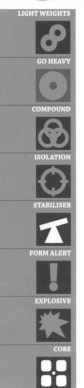
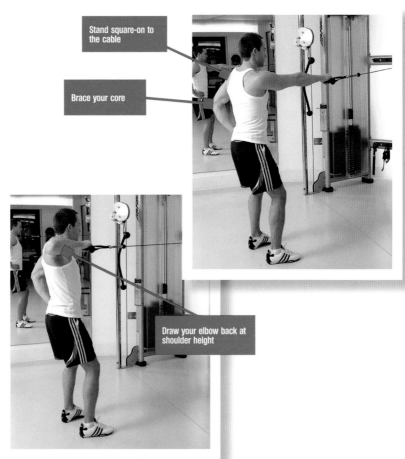

Stand square-on to the cable

Brace your core

Draw your elbow back at shoulder height

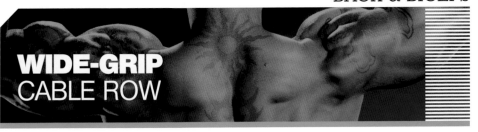

WIDE-GRIP
CABLE ROW

31

Use a long bar to shift the emphasis away from your lats and to your traps and rhomboids.

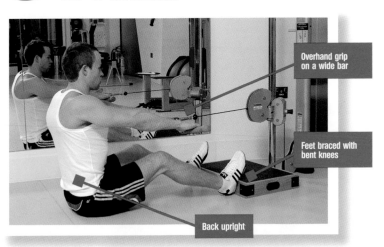

Overhand grip on a wide bar

Feet braced with bent knees

Back upright

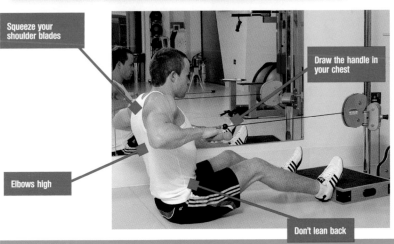

Squeeze your shoulder blades

Draw the handle in your chest

Elbows high

Don't lean back

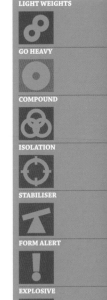

LIGHT WEIGHTS

GO HEAVY

COMPOUND

ISOLATION

STABILISER

FORM ALERT

EXPLOSIVE

CORE

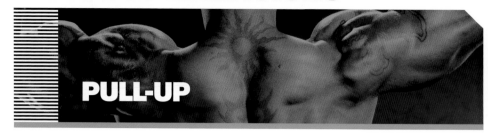

PULL-UP

32

A great test of your upper-body strength, the pull-up should be a regular in any man's gym programme. If you struggle to perform pull-ups, use a bench to help get you into the 'up' position and then lower your weight slowly.

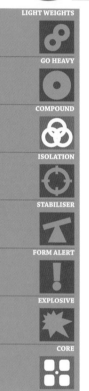

LIGHT WEIGHTS

GO HEAVY

COMPOUND

ISOLATION

STABILISER

FORM ALERT

EXPLOSIVE

CORE

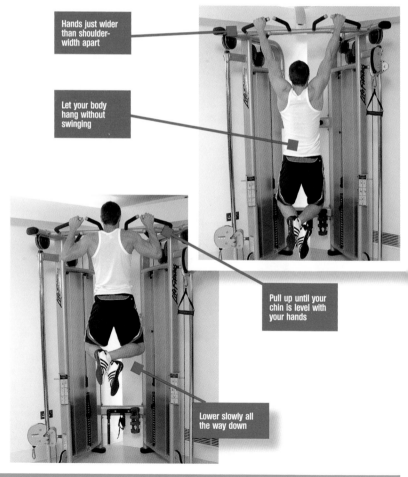

Hands just wider than shoulder-width apart

Let your body hang without swinging

Pull up until your chin is level with your hands

Lower slowly all the way down

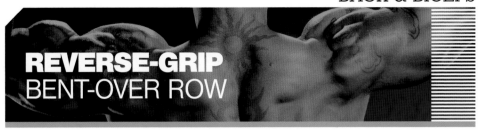

REVERSE-GRIP
BENT-OVER ROW

33

By turning your hands to face outwards you transfer the emphasis to your biceps and lats. You may find you have to reduce the weight you would use on normal bent-over rows.

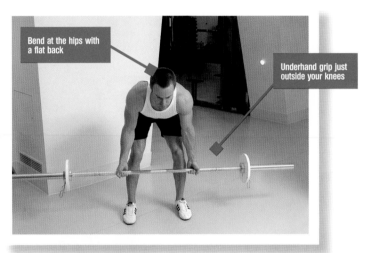

Bend at the hips with a flat back

Underhand grip just outside your knees

Squeeze your shoulder blades together

Keep your body position the same throughout

Pull the bar in to your sternum

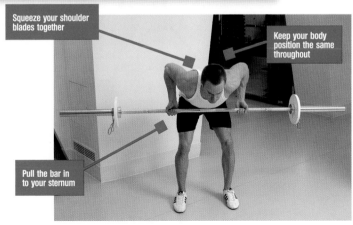

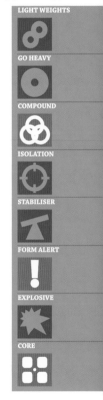

LIGHT WEIGHTS

GO HEAVY

COMPOUND

ISOLATION

STABILISER

FORM ALERT

EXPLOSIVE

CORE

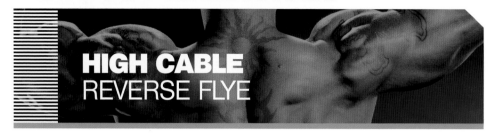

HIGH CABLE
REVERSE FLYE

34

Your rear deltoids rarely get a look-in, but adding this exercise to the mix will ensure you get balanced gains and prevent you getting hunched from having over-strong front delts that pull your shoulders forward.

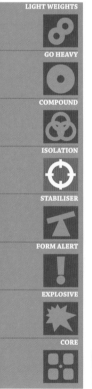

LIGHT WEIGHTS

GO HEAVY

COMPOUND

ISOLATION

STABILISER

FORM ALERT

EXPLOSIVE

CORE

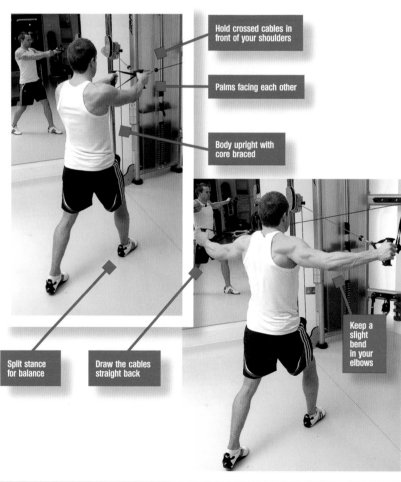

Hold crossed cables in front of your shoulders

Palms facing each other

Body upright with core braced

Split stance for balance

Draw the cables straight back

Keep a slight bend in your elbows

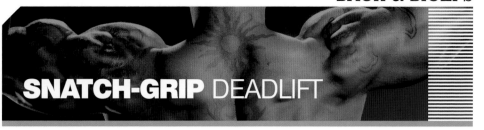

SNATCH-GRIP DEADLIFT

35

A powerful, muscle-building move that works the whole body. By taking a wide grip you make your back do more work to stabilise the bar as you lift.

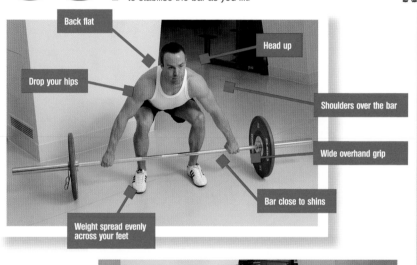

Back flat

Head up

Drop your hips

Shoulders over the bar

Wide overhand grip

Bar close to shins

Weight spread evenly across your feet

Stand up, initiating the move with your glutes

Pull your shoulders back

Push your hips forward as you stand

Keep your core braced throughout the move

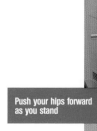

LIGHT WEIGHTS

GO HEAVY

COMPOUND

ISOLATION

STABILISER

FORM ALERT

EXPLOSIVE

CORE

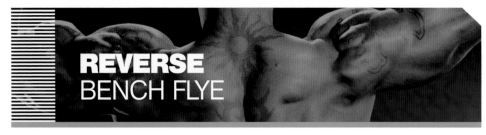

REVERSE
BENCH FLYE

36

This exercise targets the muscles of your middle back – your traps and rhomboids – while minimising the contribution from your arms.

LIGHT WEIGHTS

GO HEAVY

COMPOUND

ISOLATION

STABILISER

FORM ALERT

EXPLOSIVE

CORE

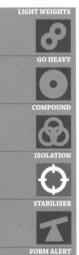

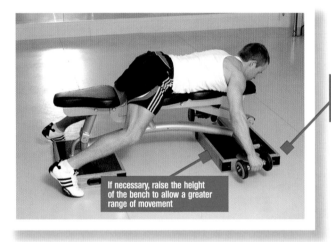

Let weights hang beneath your shoulders

If necessary, raise the height of the bench to allow a greater range of movement

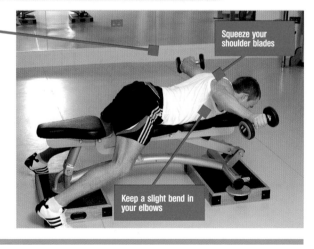

Lift your arms straight out to the sides

Squeeze your shoulder blades

Keep a slight bend in your elbows

WIDE-GRIP PULL-UP

37

Make your lats work harder by taking a wider grip on the pull-up bar. This will restrict your range of movement, but you should still aim to get your chin to hand-level and lower all the way down to complete a full rep.

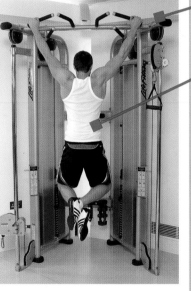

Wide overhand grip

Let your body hang without swinging

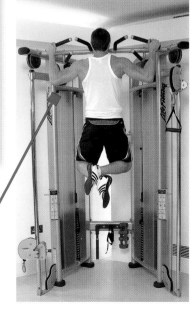

Pull up as far as you can and lower slowly all the way down

LIGHT WEIGHTS

GO HEAVY

COMPOUND

ISOLATION

STABILISER

FORM ALERT

EXPLOSIVE

CORE

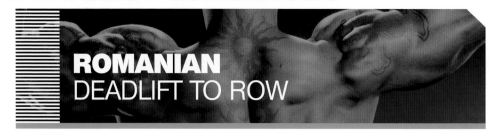

ROMANIAN
DEADLIFT TO ROW

38

This combination move gives you two classic mass-building exercises in one. You will need to keep your core braced and back straight throughout to avoid placing stress on your lower back.

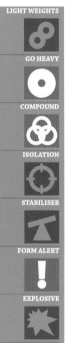

LIGHT WEIGHTS

GO HEAVY

COMPOUND

ISOLATION

STABILISER

FORM ALERT

EXPLOSIVE

CORE

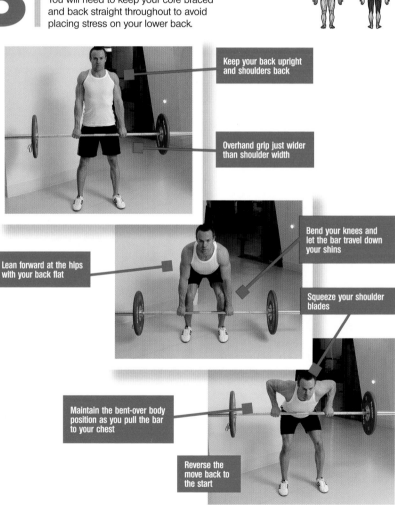

Keep your back upright and shoulders back

Overhand grip just wider than shoulder width

Bend your knees and let the bar travel down your shins

Lean forward at the hips with your back flat

Squeeze your shoulder blades

Maintain the bent-over body position as you pull the bar to your chest

Reverse the move back to the start

CLEAN
AND PRESS

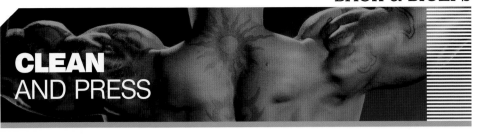

39

This exercise will work your entire body from calves to shoulders, making you functionally stronger and flooding your system with muscle-building hormones. It should be performed powerfully but with complete control, ensuring a straight back throughout.

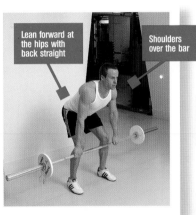

Lean forward at the hips with back straight

Shoulders over the bar

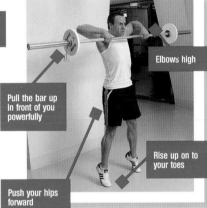

Elbows high

Pull the bar up in front of you powerfully

Rise up on to your toes

Push your hips forward

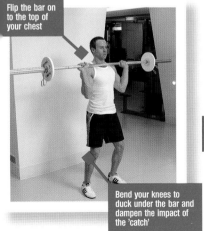

Flip the bar on to the top of your chest

Bend your knees to duck under the bar and dampen the impact of the 'catch'

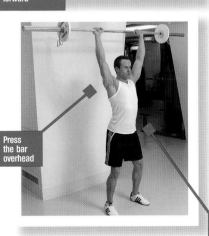

Press the bar overhead

Core braced throughout

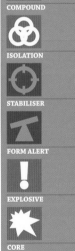

LIGHT WEIGHTS

GO HEAVY

COMPOUND

ISOLATION

STABILISER

FORM ALERT

EXPLOSIVE

CORE

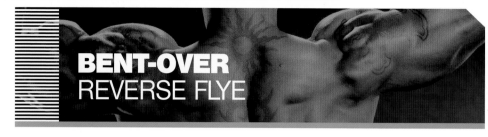

BENT-OVER
REVERSE FLYE

40

Really squeeze your shoulder blades together at the top of this move to ensure that you are working your back to the full and not just your rear shoulders.

LIGHT WEIGHTS

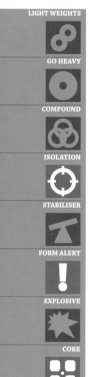

GO HEAVY

COMPOUND

ISOLATION

STABILISER

FORM ALERT

EXPLOSIVE

CORE

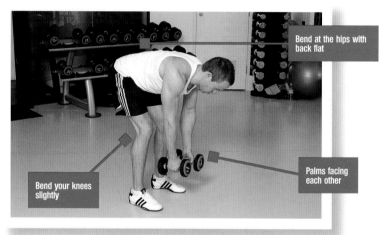

Bend at the hips with back flat

Bend your knees slightly

Palms facing each other

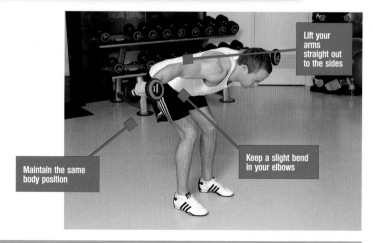

Lift your arms straight out to the sides

Maintain the same body position

Keep a slight bend in your elbows

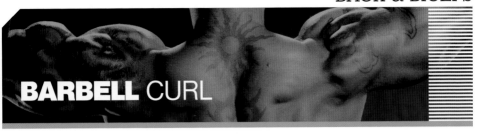

BARBELL CURL

41

This is the simplest move for packing muscle on your biceps. Pick the heaviest weight you can manage – but only with perfect form. If you have to rock your body or limit your range of motion to lift the bar, pick a lighter weight.

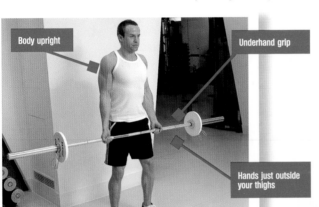

Body upright

Underhand grip

Hands just outside your thighs

Squeeze your biceps at the top of the move

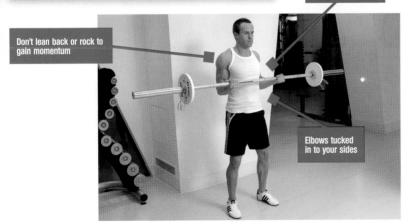

Don't lean back or rock to gain momentum

Elbows tucked in to your sides

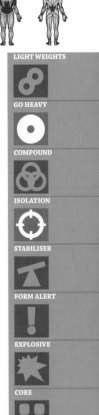

LIGHT WEIGHTS

GO HEAVY

COMPOUND

ISOLATION

STABILISER

FORM ALERT

EXPLOSIVE

CORE

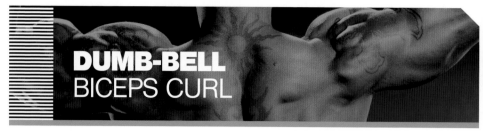

DUMB-BELL
BICEPS CURL

42

With dumb-bells you can't shift as much weight as with a bar, but you can train each arm separately, so your stronger arm can't take over the workload. By supinating your wrists – turning them out – at the top of the move you will get a greater contraction on the biceps.

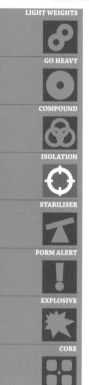

LIGHT WEIGHTS

GO HEAVY

COMPOUND

ISOLATION

STABILISER

FORM ALERT

EXPLOSIVE

CORE

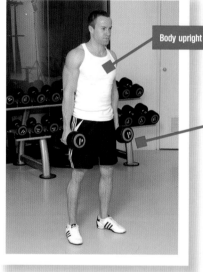

Body upright

Dumb-bells by sides, palms facing in

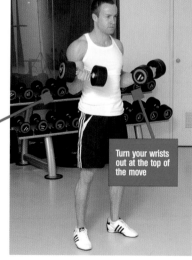

Elbows tucked in to sides

Turn your wrists out at the top of the move

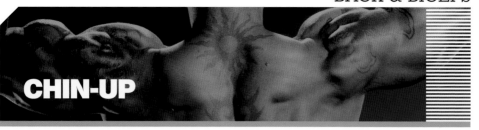

CHIN-UP

43

Use an underhand grip to place more emphasis on your biceps compared with a standard pull-up.

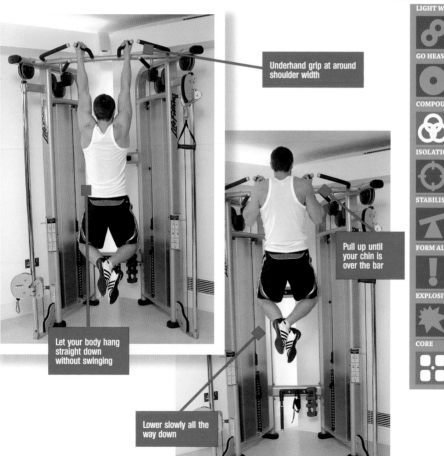

Underhand grip at around shoulder width

Let your body hang straight down without swinging

Pull up until your chin is over the bar

Lower slowly all the way down

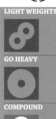

LIGHT WEIGHTS

GO HEAVY

COMPOUND

ISOLATION

STABILISER

FORM ALERT

EXPLOSIVE

CORE

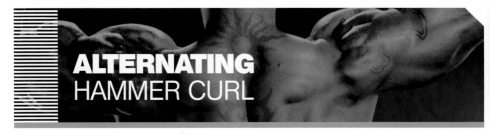

ALTERNATING
HAMMER CURL

44

The hammer grip – with palms facing each other – takes some of the pressure off your biceps brachii and places it onto your brachioradialis muscle that runs down to your forearm.

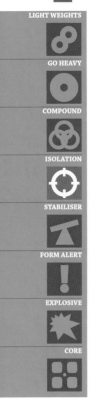

LIGHT WEIGHTS

GO HEAVY

COMPOUND

ISOLATION

STABILISER

FORM ALERT

EXPLOSIVE

CORE

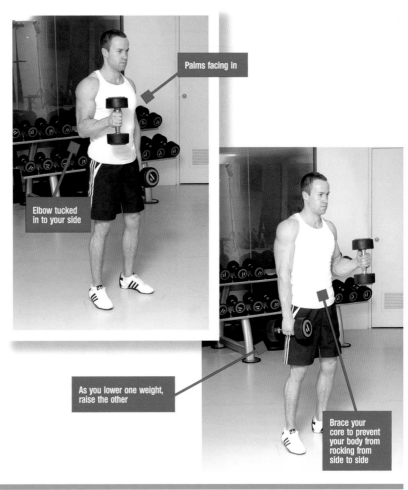

Palms facing in

Elbow tucked in to your side

As you lower one weight, raise the other

Brace your core to prevent your body from rocking from side to side

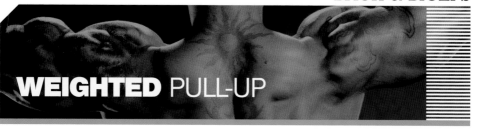

WEIGHTED PULL-UP

45

When you can perform more than ten or 12 pull-ups easily, rather than simply doing more reps, your muscles will respond better if you add extra resistance. You can hang weights from a belt or grasp a dumb-bell between your feet.

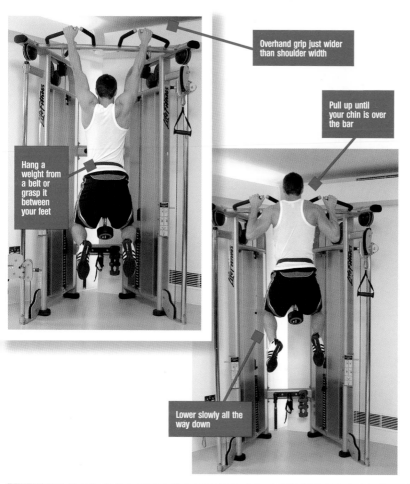

Overhand grip just wider than shoulder width

Pull up until your chin is over the bar

Hang a weight from a belt or grasp it between your feet

Lower slowly all the way down

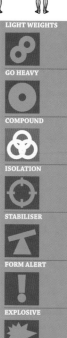

LIGHT WEIGHTS

GO HEAVY

COMPOUND

ISOLATION

STABILISER

FORM ALERT

EXPLOSIVE

CORE

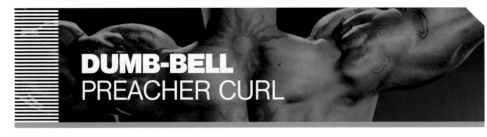

DUMB-BELL
PREACHER CURL

46

By locking your upper arm into place against the pad, you remove assistance from other muscle groups, placing all the emphasis on the biceps.

LIGHT WEIGHTS

GO HEAVY

COMPOUND

ISOLATION

STABILISER

FORM ALERT

EXPLOSIVE

CORE

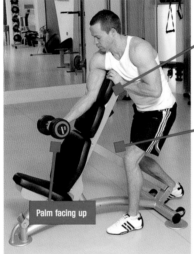

Press your upper arm against the pad

Set the bench just off the vertical

Palm facing up

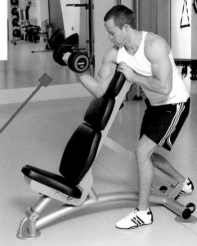

Curl the weight up without lifting your upper arm from the pad

EZ-BAR CURL

47

Like the barbell curl, this move allows you to move the maximum weight for your biceps. The zig-zag shaped EZ-bar places your palms in a more natural position than the barbell, putting less stress on your wrists and elbows.

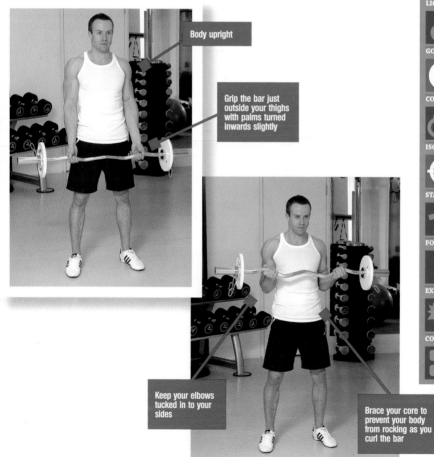

Body upright

Grip the bar just outside your thighs with palms turned inwards slightly

Keep your elbows tucked in to your sides

Brace your core to prevent your body from rocking as you curl the bar

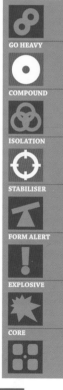

LIGHT WEIGHTS

GO HEAVY

COMPOUND

ISOLATION

STABILISER

FORM ALERT

EXPLOSIVE

CORE

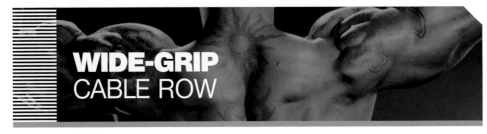

WIDE-GRIP
CABLE ROW

48

Use a long bar to shift the emphasis away from your lats and to your traps and rhomboids.

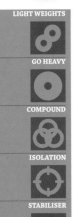

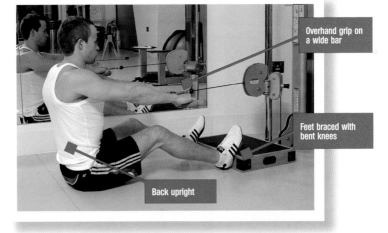

Overhand grip on a wide bar

Feet braced with bent knees

Back upright

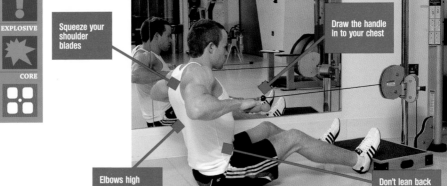

Squeeze your shoulder blades

Draw the handle in to your chest

Elbows high

Don't lean back

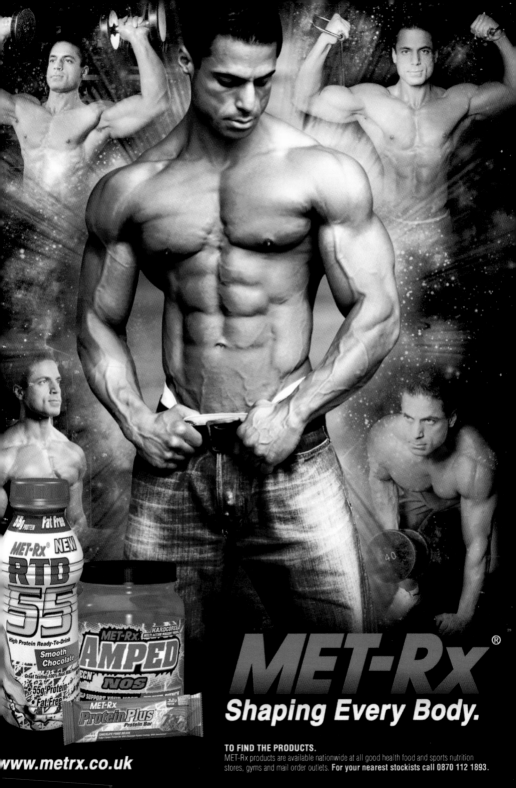

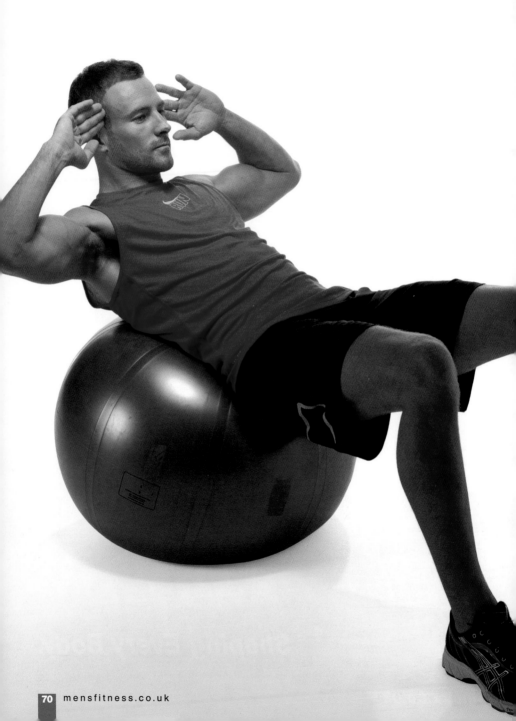

Abs & core

Your abdominals perform three main functions (or four, if you count making you look better). They stabilise your body, keeping your trunk solid when external forces are acting on it; they're responsible for forward bending and rotational movements; and they control side bending and back extension movements. These are the four main muscles in the group.

Transversus abdominis

The transverses abdominis is a deeply-lying muscle that runs across your torso from side to side, holding your ribs in place and stabilising your pelvic area.

Internal obliques

These run upwards from your hip, allowing you to bend and rotate to the sides.

External obliques

These lie above the internal obliques, and work alongside others to bend and rotate your torso.

Rectus abdominis

At the front of your stomach is your rectus abdominis – the abs. This sheet of muscle is separated into segments, giving you the classic six-pack look when it is developed.

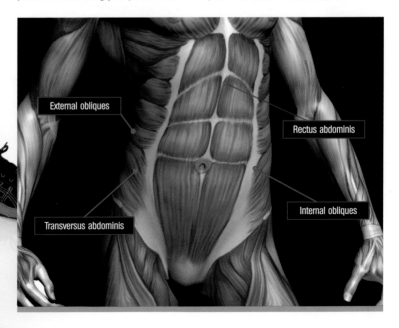

External obliques

Rectus abdominis

Transversus abdominis

Internal obliques

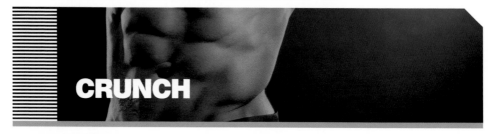

CRUNCH

49

The original abs move. Remember to keep the pace slow, especially as you lower back down, to keep the maximum tension on your stomach muscles.

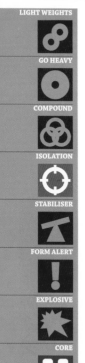

LIGHT WEIGHTS

GO HEAVY

COMPOUND

ISOLATION

STABILISER

FORM ALERT

EXPLOSIVE

CORE

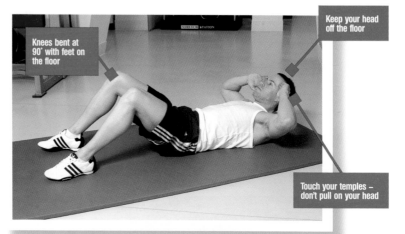

Knees bent at 90° with feet on the floor

Keep your head off the floor

Touch your temples – don't pull on your head

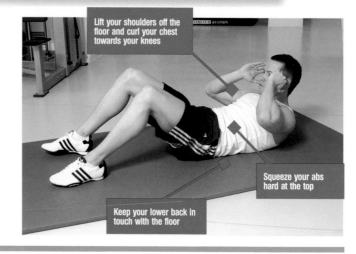

Lift your shoulders off the floor and curl your chest towards your knees

Squeeze your abs hard at the top

Keep your lower back in touch with the floor

SEATED
RUSSIAN TWIST

50

Build power for sport with a move that requires you to maintain an angled body position while twisting through your torso.

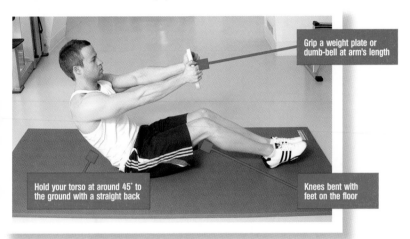

Grip a weight plate or dumb-bell at arm's length

Hold your torso at around 45° to the ground with a straight back

Knees bent with feet on the floor

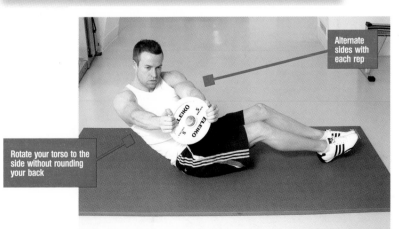

Rotate your torso to the side without rounding your back

Alternate sides with each rep

LIGHT WEIGHTS

GO HEAVY

COMPOUND

ISOLATION

STABILISER

FORM ALERT

EXPLOSIVE

CORE

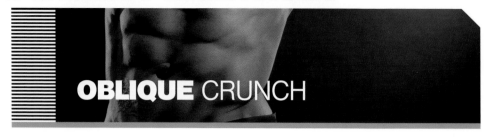

OBLIQUE CRUNCH

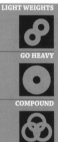

51

This move targets your side abs. Hold the 'up' position for a one-count and lower slowly again to stop momentum from doing the work.

LIGHT WEIGHTS

GO HEAVY

COMPOUND

ISOLATION

STABILISER

FORM ALERT

EXPLOSIVE

CORE

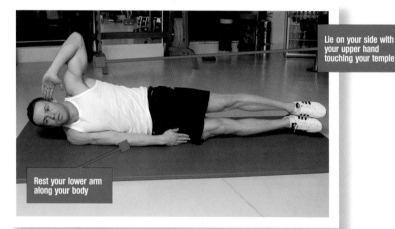

Lie on your side with your upper hand touching your temple

Rest your lower arm along your body

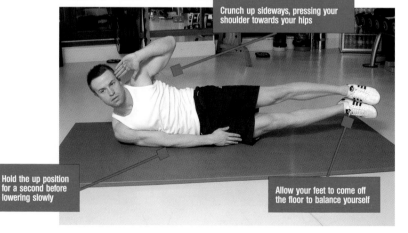

Crunch up sideways, pressing your shoulder towards your hips

Hold the up position for a second before lowering slowly

Allow your feet to come off the floor to balance yourself

REVERSE CRUNCH

52

By lifting your legs towards your chest you place most of the emphasis on the lower portion of your abs.

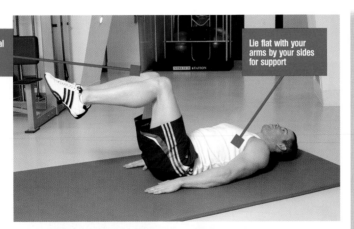

Thighs vertical with knees bent at 90°

Lie flat with your arms by your sides for support

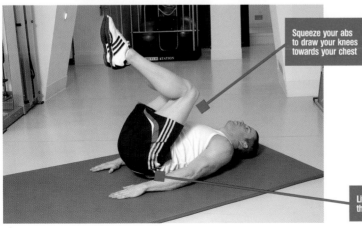

Squeeze your abs to draw your knees towards your chest

Lift your hips off the floor

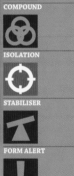

LIGHT WEIGHTS

GO HEAVY

COMPOUND

ISOLATION

STABILISER

FORM ALERT

EXPLOSIVE

CORE

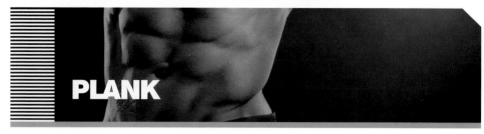

PLANK

53

This classic stability move strengthens your deep core muscles, helping to improve posture and protect your lower back from injury during heavy lifts such as squats and deadlifts.

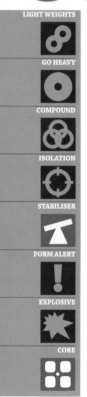

LIGHT WEIGHTS

GO HEAVY

COMPOUND

ISOLATION

STABILISER

FORM ALERT

EXPLOSIVE

CORE

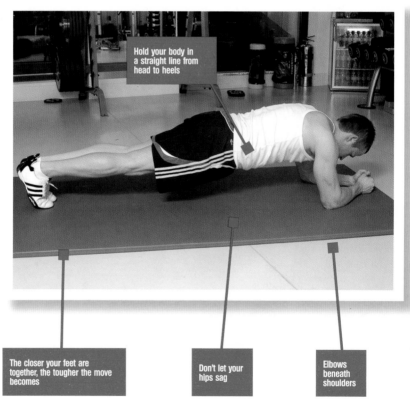

Hold your body in a straight line from head to heels

The closer your feet are together, the tougher the move becomes

Don't let your hips sag

Elbows beneath shoulders

GYM BALL CRUNCH

54

As well as providing an unstable surface that trains your deep stabiliser muscles, the gym ball also allows you to get a greater range of motion over the standard crunch, giving your abs a better workout.

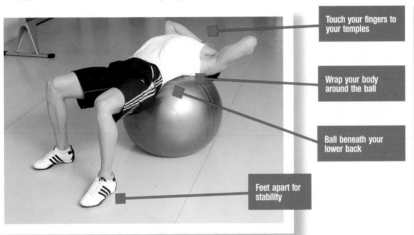

Touch your fingers to your temples

Wrap your body around the ball

Ball beneath your lower back

Feet apart for stability

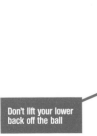

Use your abs to pull your shoulders up as much as possible

Don't lift your lower back off the ball

Hold the up position for a second before lowering slowly

LIGHT WEIGHTS

GO HEVY

COMPOUND

ISOLATION

STABILISER

FORM ALERT

EXPLOSIVE

CORE

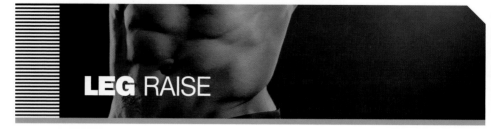

LEG RAISE

55

This move can be tough, not least because you have to hang from the bar for the duration of each set. If you raise just your legs, you'll mainly be working your hip flexor muscles rather than your abs, so aim to draw your knees to your chest to work your abs hard.

LIGHT WEIGHTS

GO HEAVY

COMPOUND

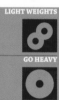

ISOLATION

STABILISER

FORM ALERT

EXPLOSIVE

CORE

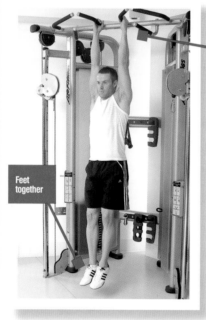

Feet together

Hang from a pull-up bar (some gyms provide elbow straps if you find it hard to hang on for the full set)

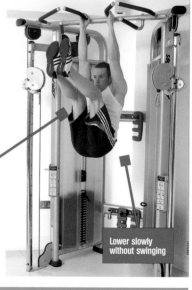

Use your abs to draw your knees to your chest

Lower slowly without swinging

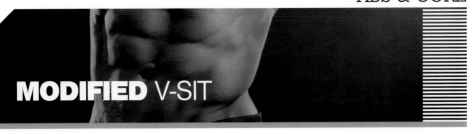

MODIFIED V-SIT

56

This requires a certain amount of balance and co-ordination because you need to keep your weight centred over your glutes to avoid falling forwards or backwards.

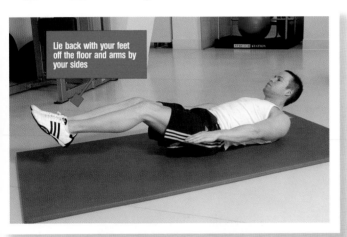

Lie back with your feet off the floor and arms by your sides

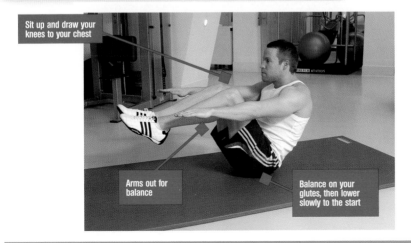

Sit up and draw your knees to your chest

Arms out for balance

Balance on your glutes, then lower slowly to the start

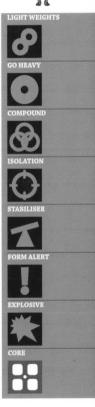

LIGHT WEIGHTS

GO HEAVY

COMPOUND

ISOLATION

STABILISER

FORM ALERT

EXPLOSIVE

CORE

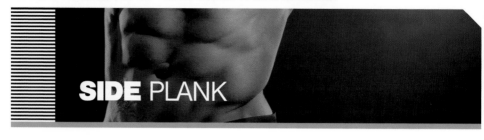

SIDE PLANK

57

Like the standard plank, this exercise trains the deep core muscles to help stabilise your spine during heavy lifts and sporting movements.

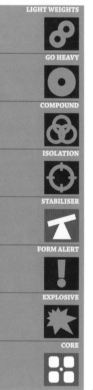

LIGHT WEIGHTS

GO HEAVY

COMPOUND

ISOLATION

STABILISER

FORM ALERT

EXPLOSIVE

CORE

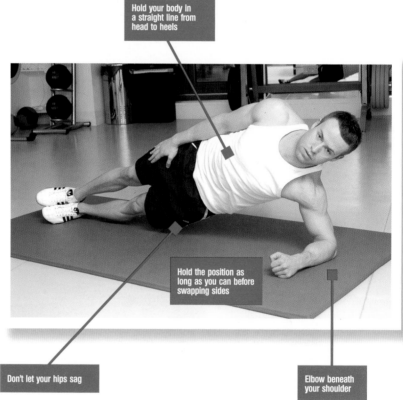

Hold your body in a straight line from head to heels

Hold the position as long as you can before swapping sides

Don't let your hips sag

Elbow beneath your shoulder

WEIGHTED CRUNCH

58

By holding a weight plate or dumb-bell across your chest when doing crunches, you can adjust the resistance so that you get near to failure within the muscle-building ten-to-12 rep range.

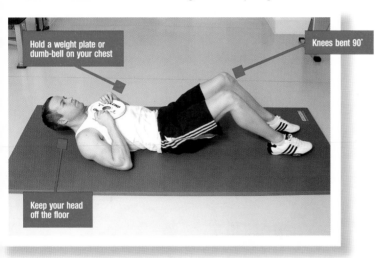

Hold a weight plate or dumb-bell on your chest

Knees bent 90°

Keep your head off the floor

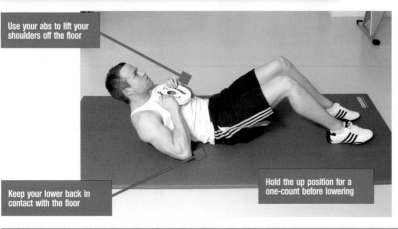

Use your abs to lift your shoulders off the floor

Keep your lower back in contact with the floor

Hold the up position for a one-count before lowering

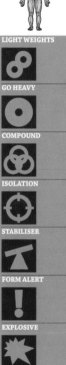

LIGHT WEIGHTS

GO HEAVY

COMPOUND

ISOLATION

STABILISER

FORM ALERT

EXPLOSIVE

CORE

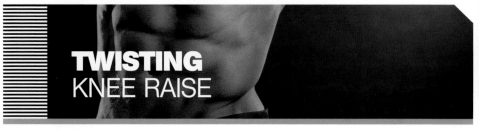

TWISTING KNEE RAISE

59

Pull your knees up to the sides to give your side abs (obliques) a workout. The straighter your legs, the tougher the exercise.

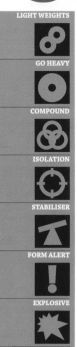

LIGHT WEIGHTS

GO HEAVY

COMPOUND

ISOLATION

STABILISER

FORM ALERT

EXPLOSIVE

CORE

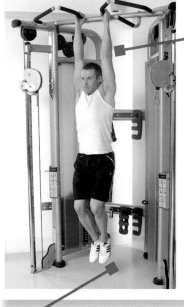

Hang from a pull-up bar without swinging

Feet together

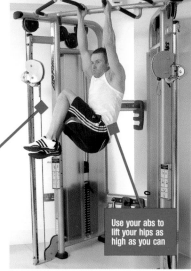

Draw your knees up and to the side

Use your abs to lift your hips as high as you can

GYM BALL
OBLIQUE CRUNCH

60

The gym ball lets you get a greater range of motion on this move. Press your feet against a wall to hold your body on the ball.

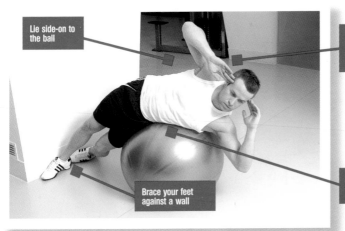

Lie side-on to the ball

Touch your hands to your temples

Brace your feet against a wall

Ball beneath your hips

LIGHT WEIGHTS

GO HEAVY

COMPOUND

ISOLATION

STABILISER

FORM ALERT

EXPLOSIVE

CORE

Engage your side abs to lift your body up

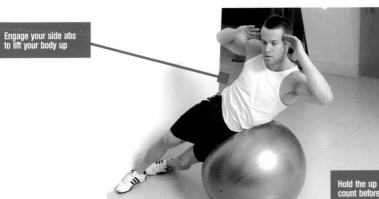

Hold the up position for a one-count before lowering slowly

STANDING CABLE
RUSSIAN TWIST

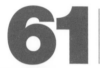

61 The cable keeps a constant tension on your muscles, developing core power for sports that require twisting and throwing movements.

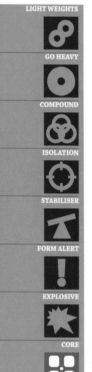

LIGHT WEIGHTS

GO HEAVY

COMPOUND

ISOLATION

STABILISER

FORM ALERT

EXPLOSIVE

CORE

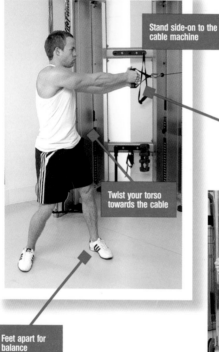

Stand side-on to the cable machine

Stand far enough from the cable to ensure that it is under tension at all times

Twist your torso towards the cable

Feet apart for balance

Arms straight at chest height

Twist your torso as far as you can while keeping your back straight

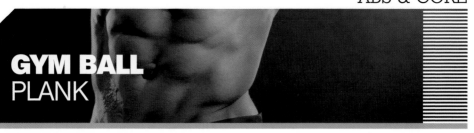

GYM BALL
PLANK

62

Preventing the ball from wobbling requires strong core muscles. Aim to increase the time you hold the plank by ten seconds each time you try it.

The closer your feet are together, the harder the move becomes

Shoulders directly over your elbows

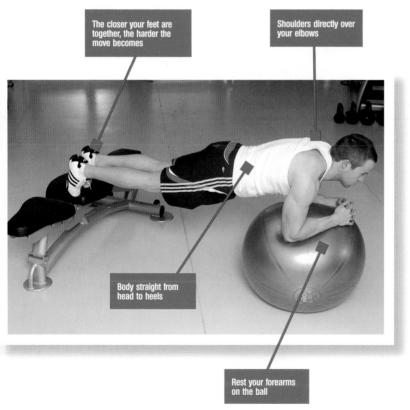

Body straight from head to heels

Rest your forearms on the ball

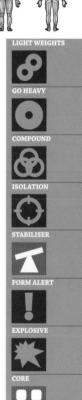

LIGHT WEIGHTS

GO HEAVY

COMPOUND

ISOLATION

STABILISER

FORM ALERT

EXPLOSIVE

CORE

101 BEST EXERCISES

MEDICINE BALL
KNEE RAISE

63

Adding resistance to this tough move will limit the number of reps you can perform, giving your abs a muscle-building stimulus.

LIGHT WEIGHTS

GO HEAVY

COMPOUND

ISOLATION

STABILISER

FORM ALERT

EXPLOSIVE

CORE

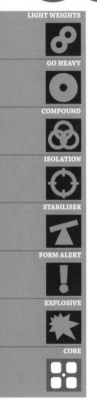

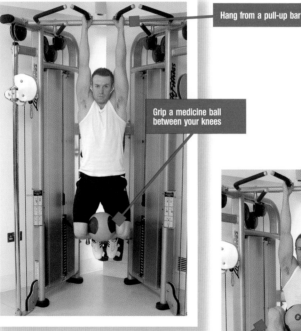

Hang from a pull-up bar

Grip a medicine ball between your knees

Draw your knees up to your chest

Use your abs to lift your hips as much as possible

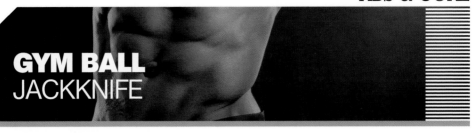

GYM BALL
JACKKNIFE

64

Keep your hips high and crunch your hips towards your chest to work your abs. If you just pull your knees back and forth then you will mainly work your hip flexors, not your abs.

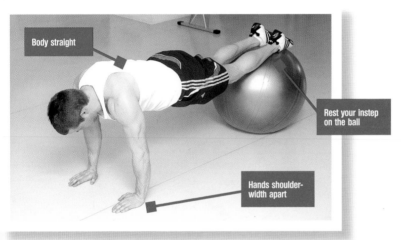

Body straight

Rest your instep on the ball

Hands shoulder-width apart

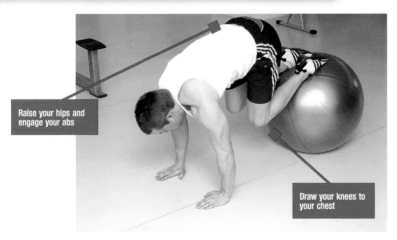

Raise your hips and engage your abs

Draw your knees to your chest

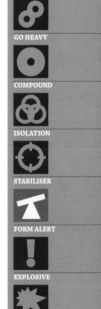

LIGHT WEIGHTS

GO HEAVY

COMPOUND

ISOLATION

STABILISER

FORM ALERT

EXPLOSIVE

CORE

LOWER-BODY
RUSSIAN TWIST

65

Place the emphasis on your lower core muscles by transferring the twisting movement to your lower body, while keeping your shoulders flat on the floor.

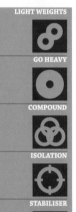

LIGHT WEIGHTS

GO HEAVY

COMPOUND

ISOLATION

STABILISER

FORM ALERT

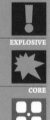

EXPLOSIVE

CORE

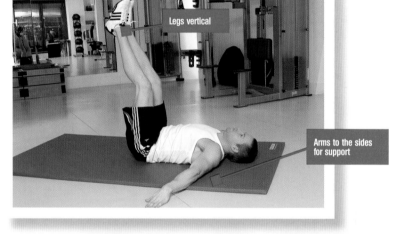

Legs vertical

Arms to the sides for support

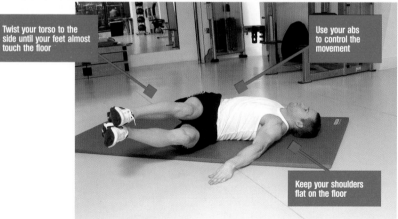

Twist your torso to the side until your feet almost touch the floor

Use your abs to control the movement

Keep your shoulders flat on the floor

GYM BALL
PASSING JACKKNIFE

66 Passing the ball from hands to feet, and back again, forces you to perform the jackknife movement correctly and under control.

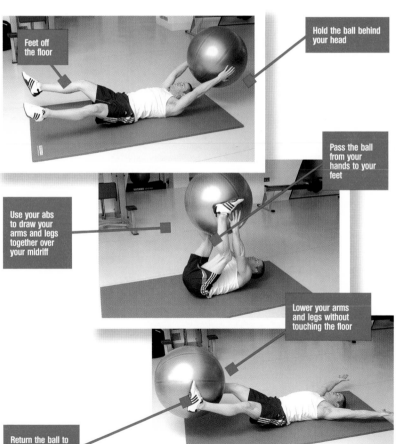

Hold the ball behind your head

Feet off the floor

Pass the ball from your hands to your feet

Use your abs to draw your arms and legs together over your midriff

Lower your arms and legs without touching the floor

Return the ball to your hands on the following rep

LIGHT WEIGHTS

GO HEAVY

COMPOUND

ISOLATION

STABILISER

FORM ALERT

EXPLOSIVE

CORE

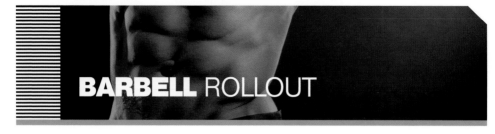

BARBELL ROLLOUT

67

Use your core muscles to control the movement slowly up and down without letting your hips sag.

LIGHT WEIGHTS

GO HEAVY

COMPOUND

ISOLATION

STABILISER

FORM ALERT

EXPLOSIVE

CORE

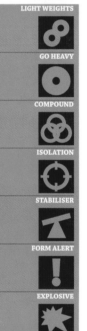

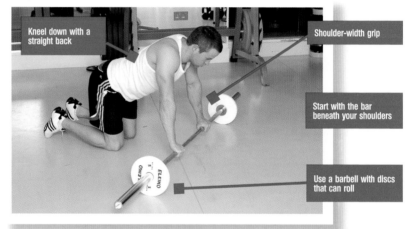

Kneel down with a straight back

Shoulder-width grip

Start with the bar beneath your shoulders

Use a barbell with discs that can roll

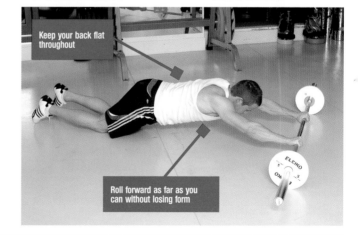

Keep your back flat throughout

Roll forward as far as you can without losing form

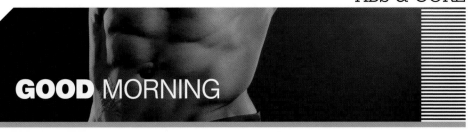

GOOD MORNING

68

Keep the weight light when you first try this exercise to prevent possible strain to your lower back.

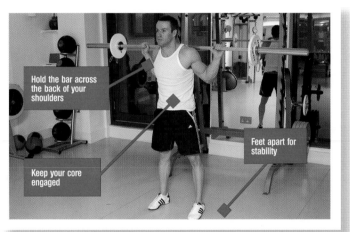

Hold the bar across the back of your shoulders

Keep your core engaged

Feet apart for stability

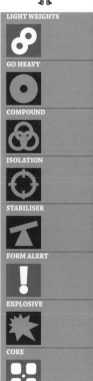

LIGHT WEIGHTS

GO HEAVY

COMPOUND

ISOLATION

STABILISER

FORM ALERT

EXPLOSIVE

CORE

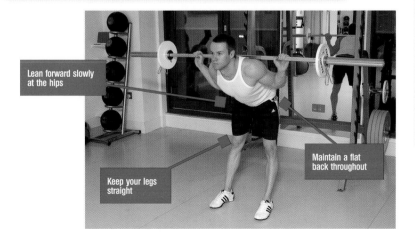

Lean forward slowly at the hips

Keep your legs straight

Maintain a flat back throughout

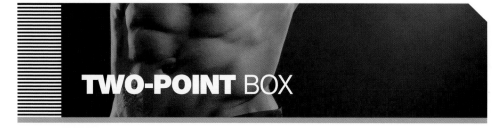

TWO-POINT BOX

69

Build your spine's supporting muscles to aid posture.

LIGHT WEIGHTS

GO HEAVY

COMPOUND

ISOLATION

STABILISER

FORM ALERT

EXPLOSIVE

CORE

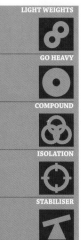

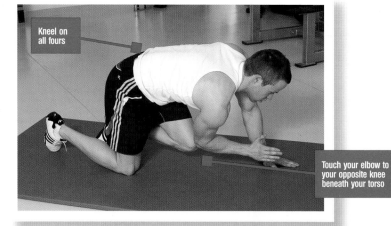

Kneel on all fours

Touch your elbow to your opposite knee beneath your torso

Extend your arm and leg until they form a straight line with your body

Hold the position for a two-count before repeating

MEDICINE BALL
SLEDGEHAMMER

70 Perform this exercise explosively, using your core muscles to control the movement.

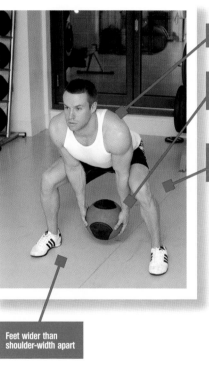

Back flat

Hold a medicine ball between your legs

Bend at the hips and knees

Stand up and raise the ball over your head

Feet wider than shoulder-width apart

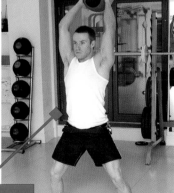

Bring the ball down powerfully, using your abs to control the movement

LIGHT WEIGHTS

GO HEAVY

COMPOUND

ISOLATION

STABILISER

FORM ALERT

EXPLOSIVE

CORE

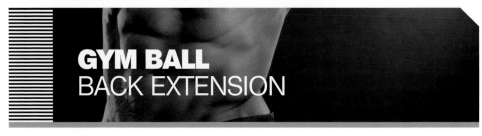

GYM BALL
BACK EXTENSION

71

Using a gym ball allows you to get a full range of motion on this classic lower-back exercise, while the additional wobble works the deep stabilising muscles in your core.

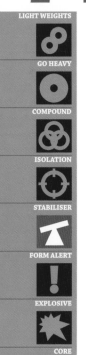

LIGHT WEIGHTS

GO HEAVY

COMPOUND

ISOLATION

STABILISER

FORM ALERT

EXPLOSIVE

CORE

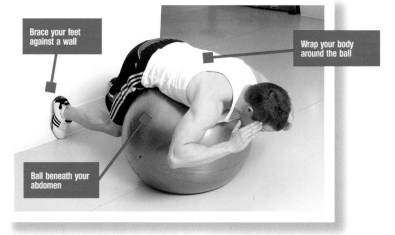

Brace your feet against a wall

Wrap your body around the ball

Ball beneath your abdomen

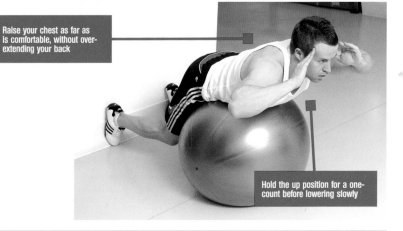

Raise your chest as far as is comfortable, without over-extending your back

Hold the up position for a one-count before lowering slowly

WOODCHOP

72

This exercise requires your whole body to work through several planes of motion at the same time – lifting and rotating simultaneously – using your core muscles to control the transfer of power from your lower body to upper.

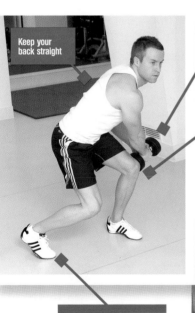

Keep your back straight

Hold the dumb-bell to the outside of your thigh

Bend at the knees and hips

Bring the weight up and across your body

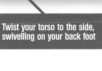

Twist your torso to the side, swivelling on your back foot

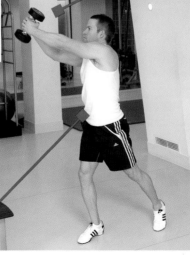

Use your core muscles to control the motion

LIGHT WEIGHTS

GO HEAVY

COMPOUND

ISOLATION

STABILISER

FORM ALERT

EXPLOSIVE

CORE

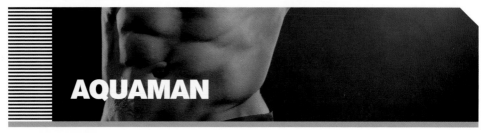

AQUAMAN

73

The swimming motion with your hands and feet strengthens the muscles that support your spine during dynamic sporting movements.

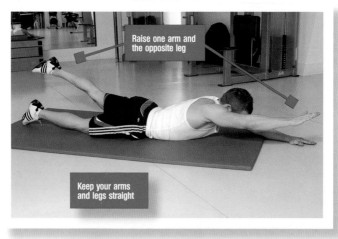

Raise one arm and the opposite leg

Keep your arms and legs straight

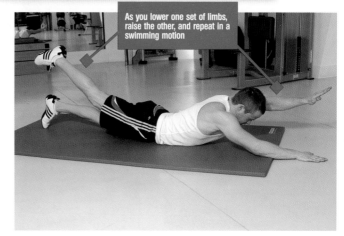

As you lower one set of limbs, raise the other, and repeat in a swimming motion

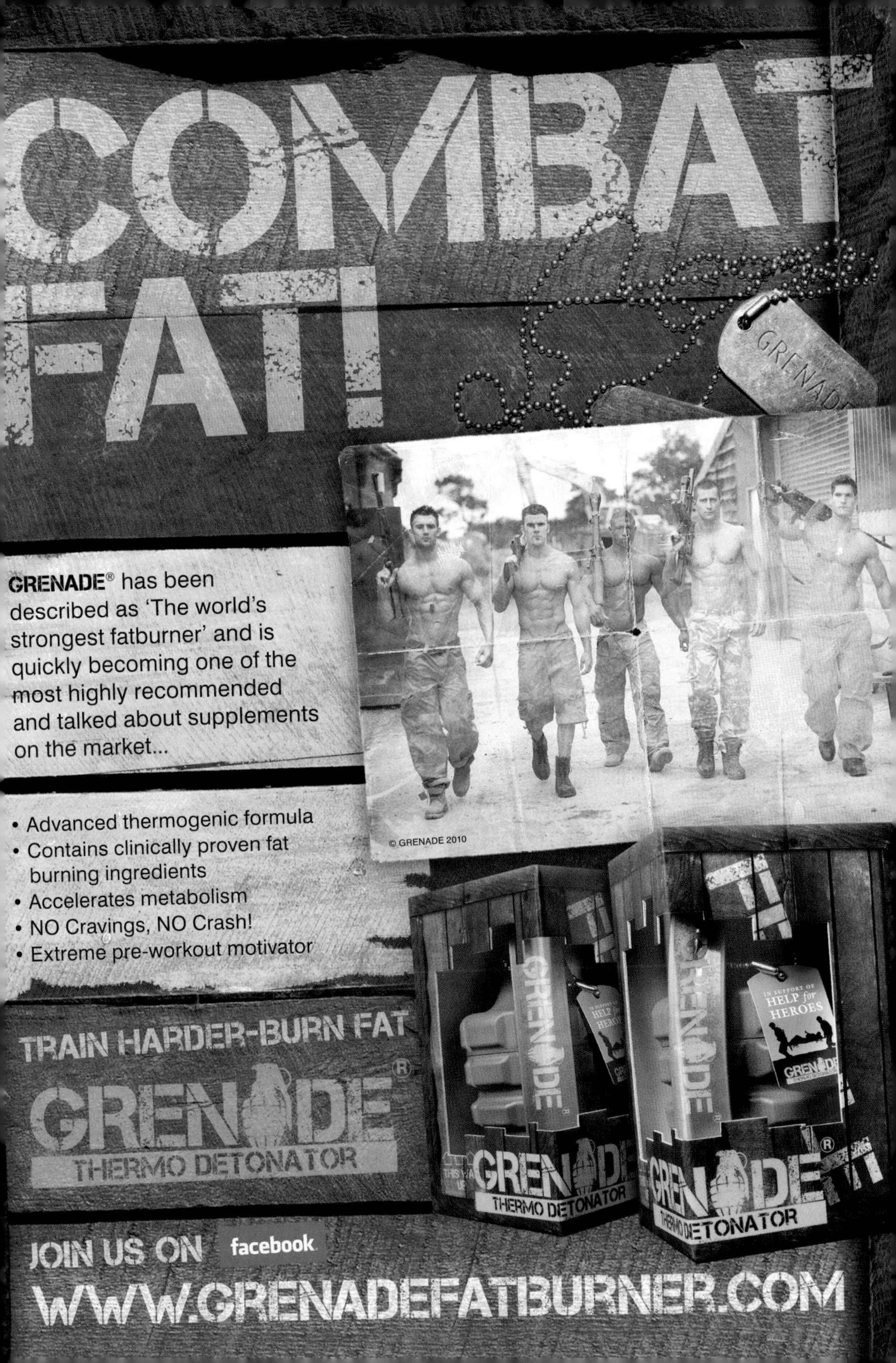

COMBAT FAT!
GRENADE
GRENADE® has been described as 'The world's strongest fatburner' and is quickly becoming one of the most highly recommended and talked about supplements on the market...
© GRENADE 2010
• Advanced thermogenic formula
• Contains clinically proven fat burning ingredients
• Accelerates metabolism
• NO Cravings, NO Crash!
• Extreme pre-workout motivator
TRAIN HARDER-BURN FAT
GRENADE®
THERMO DETONATOR
IN SUPPORT OF HELP for HEROES
GRENADE
THERMO DETONATOR
JOIN US ON facebook
WWW.GRENADEFATBURNER.COM

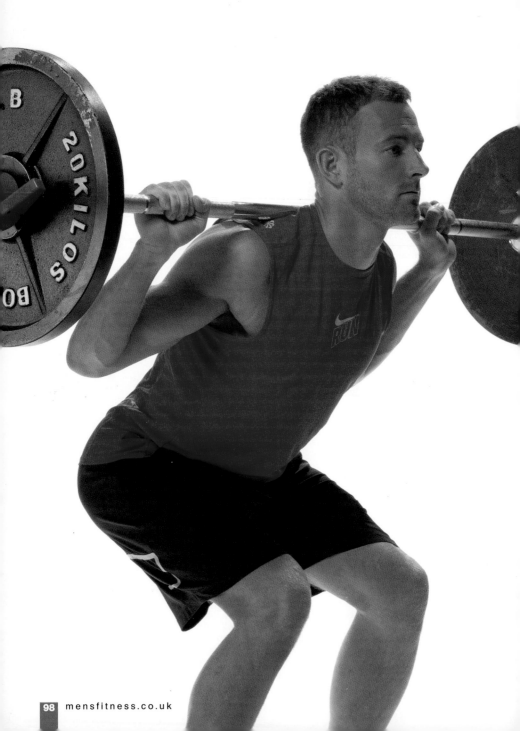

Legs

Your legs and backside (glutes) contain the biggest muscles in your body and they make up about half your total muscle mass. Training the lower half of your body will have a positive impact on the upper half because training these large muscles provokes a huge growth hormone response.

On the front of your thighs the quads help straighten your leg and stabilise your knee. On the back of your thigh your hamstrings are responsible for extending your hips and bending your knees. Both these muscle groups work with your glutes every time you go from a sitting to a standing position.

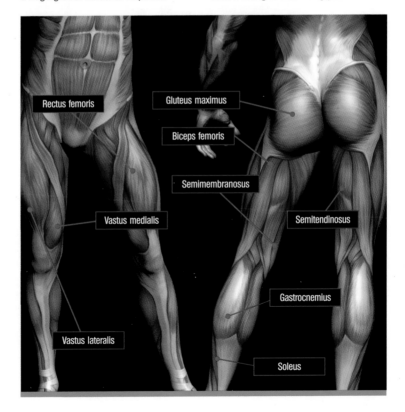

Rectus femoris

Gluteus maximus

Biceps femoris

Semimembranosus

Vastus medialis

Semitendinosus

Gastrocnemius

Vastus lateralis

Soleus

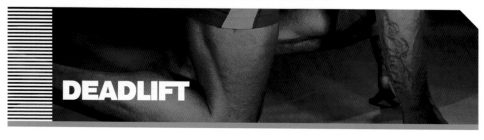

DEADLIFT

74

The original power move. The deadlift uses several large muscle groups, which floods your body with muscle-building hormones.

LIGHT WEIGHTS

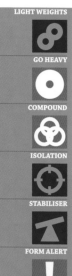

GO HEAVY

COMPOUND

ISOLATION

STABILISER

FORM ALERT

EXPLOSIVE

CORE

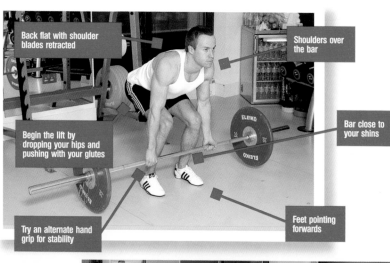

Back flat with shoulder blades retracted

Shoulders over the bar

Begin the lift by dropping your hips and pushing with your glutes

Bar close to your shins

Try an alternate hand grip for stability

Feet pointing forwards

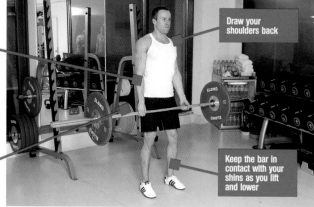

Keep your core muscles contracted throughout the lift

Draw your shoulders back

Push your hips forward

Keep the bar in contact with your shins as you lift and lower

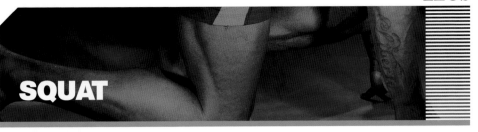

SQUAT

75

The squat is a classic move that builds muscle throughout your lower body and should form the basis of all your leg training. Some people find the squat difficult to perform well, but keep practising and perfecting your form and you'll be repaid in spades.

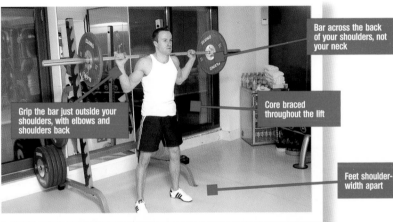

Bar across the back of your shoulders, not your neck

Grip the bar just outside your shoulders, with elbows and shoulders back

Core braced throughout the lift

Feet shoulder-width apart

Back straight

Head up

Lower until your thighs are at least horizontal

Your feet should point in the same direction as your knees

LIGHT WEIGHTS

GO HEAVY

COMPOUND

ISOLATION

STABILISER

FORM ALERT

EXPLOSIVE

CORE

101 BEST EXERCISES

DUMB-BELL SQUAT

76

Using dumb-bells instead of a bar can take the pressure off your lower back by allowing you to keep your torso more upright as you squat.

LIGHT WEIGHTS

GO HEAVY

COMPOUND

ISOLATION

STABILISER

FORM ALERT

EXPLOSIVE

CORE

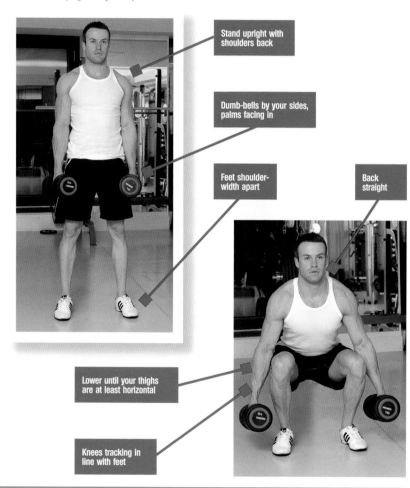

Stand upright with shoulders back

Dumb-bells by your sides, palms facing in

Feet shoulder-width apart

Back straight

Lower until your thighs are at least horizontal

Knees tracking in line with feet

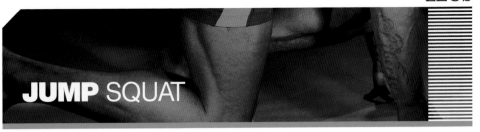

JUMP SQUAT

77

This explosive move fires up the fast-twitch muscles in your quads – the ones with the most potential for growth.

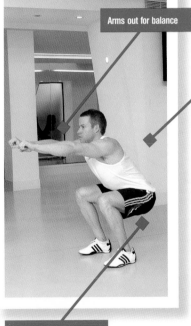

Arms out for balance

Back flat

Lower until your thighs are at least horizontal

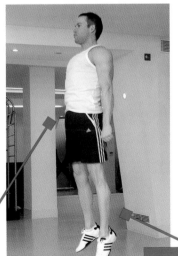

Push up powerfully and jump as high as you can

As you land, go straight into the next squat

LIGHT WEIGHTS

GO HEAVY

COMPOUND

ISOLATION

STABILISER

FORM ALERT

EXPLOSIVE

CORE

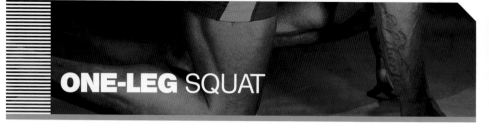

ONE-LEG SQUAT

78

Squatting on one leg strengthens the stabilising muscles in your hips, knees and ankles, giving you a more solid platform from which to increase the weight you squat, and protecting your joints from injury.

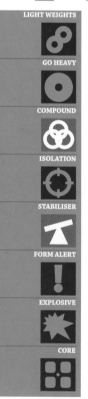

LIGHT WEIGHTS

GO HEAVY

COMPOUND

ISOLATION

STABILISER

FORM ALERT

EXPLOSIVE

CORE

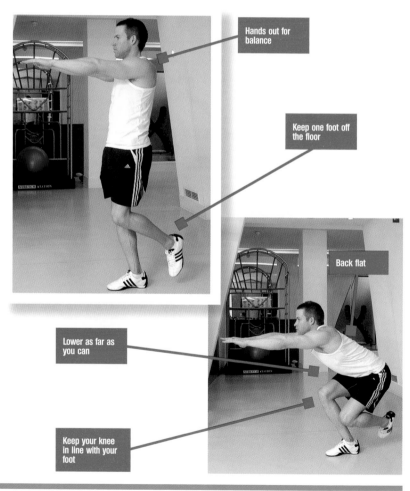

Hands out for balance

Keep one foot off the floor

Back flat

Lower as far as you can

Keep your knee in line with your foot

DUMB-BELL
GYM BALL SQUAT

79

Using a gym ball to support your back places the focus of the squat firmly on your quads.

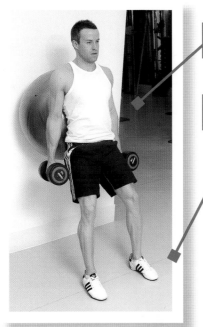

Start with the ball behind your lower back

Place your feet in front of your body

Back upright

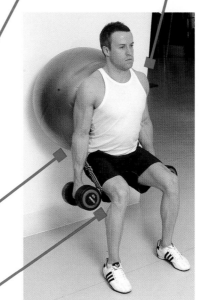

Lower slowly, rolling your back down the ball

Knees in line with feet

LIGHT WEIGHTS
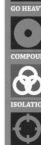

GO HEAVY

COMPOUND

ISOLATION

STABILISER

FORM ALERT
!

EXPLOSIVE

CORE

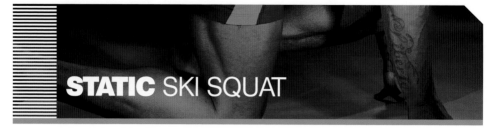

STATIC SKI SQUAT

80

This isometric (holding a position under tension) exercise will help build muscle endurance in your thighs, which will in turn allow you to lift heavier when you return to normal squats.

LIGHT WEIGHTS

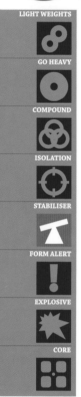

GO HEAVY

COMPOUND

ISOLATION

STABILISER

FORM ALERT

EXPLOSIVE

CORE

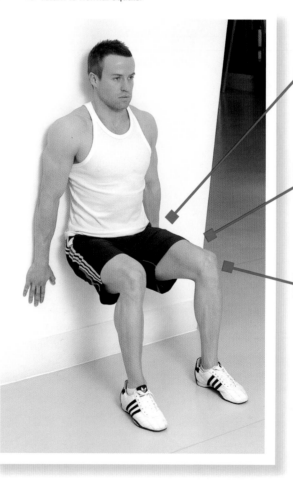

Hips and shoulders against the wall

Thighs horizontal

Knees bent 90°

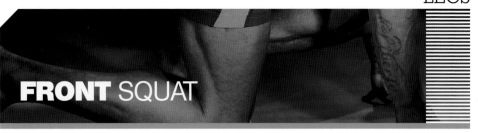

FRONT SQUAT

81

By holding the bar in front of you, as opposed to behind your neck, it naturally alters your posture so your torso is more upright. This will decrease the pressure on your lower back and place more emphasis on your quads than a standard squat does.

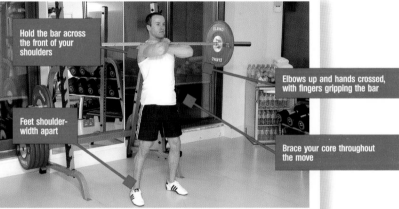

Hold the bar across the front of your shoulders

Feet shoulder-width apart

Elbows up and hands crossed, with fingers gripping the bar

Brace your core throughout the move

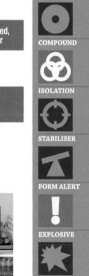

LIGHT WEIGHTS

GO HEAVY

COMPOUND

ISOLATION

STABILISER

FORM ALERT

EXPLOSIVE

CORE

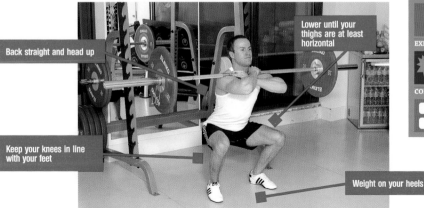

Back straight and head up

Lower until your thighs are at least horizontal

Keep your knees in line with your feet

Weight on your heels

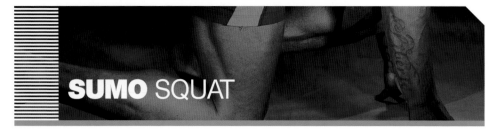

SUMO SQUAT

82

The wider stance transfers some of the stress of the squat on to your inner thighs – the adductors.

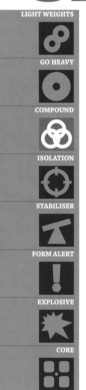

LIGHT WEIGHTS

GO HEAVY

COMPOUND

ISOLATION

STABILISER

FORM ALERT

EXPLOSIVE

CORE

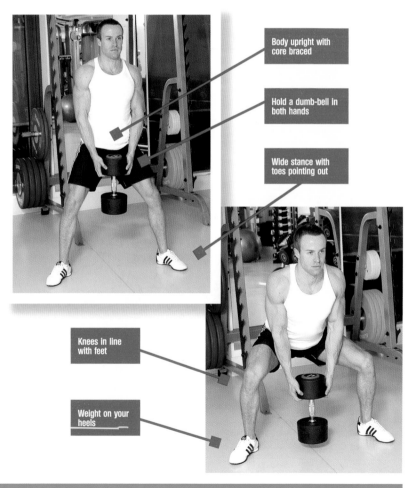

Body upright with core braced

Hold a dumb-bell in both hands

Wide stance with toes pointing out

Knees in line with feet

Weight on your heels

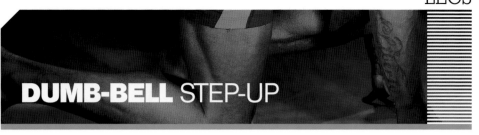

DUMB-BELL STEP-UP

83

Target your quads and glutes with a move that will help to stabilise your knee joint, making you more efficient at running.

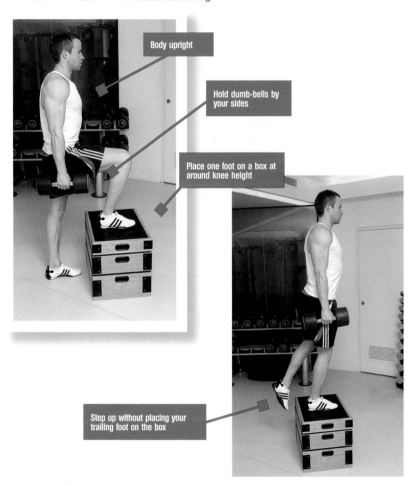

Body upright

Hold dumb-bells by your sides

Place one foot on a box at around knee height

Step up without placing your trailing foot on the box

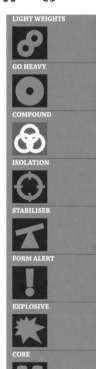

LIGHT WEIGHTS

GO HEAVY

COMPOUND

ISOLATION

STABILISER

FORM ALERT

EXPLOSIVE

CORE

101 BEST EXERCISES

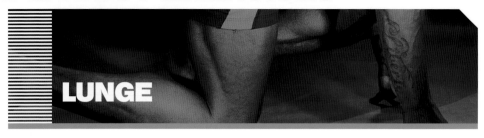

LUNGE

84

This move works your entire lower body and requires good balance and flexibility at the hip, so it will help to make you more dynamic when playing sport.

LIGHT WEIGHTS

GO HEAVY

COMPOUND

ISOLATION

STABILISER

FORM ALERT

EXPLOSIVE

CORE

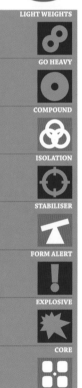

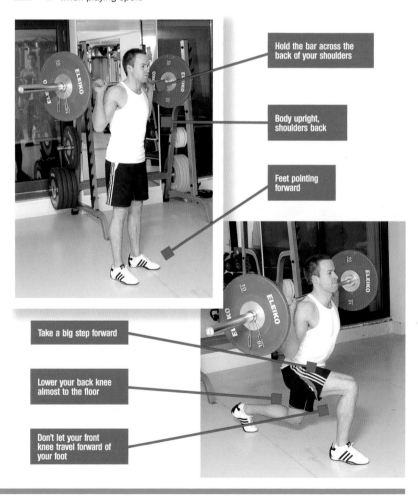

Hold the bar across the back of your shoulders

Body upright, shoulders back

Feet pointing forward

Take a big step forward

Lower your back knee almost to the floor

Don't let your front knee travel forward of your foot

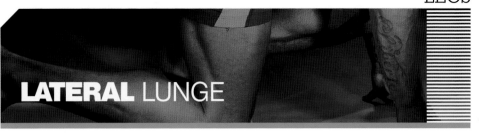

LATERAL LUNGE

85

Lunging to the side works your quads and your inner thighs. You can develop this move by lunging at different angles to stimulate your leg muscles in different ways.

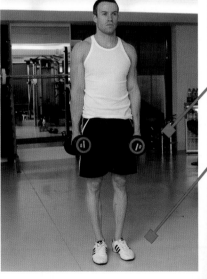

Stand upright with dumbbells by your sides

Feet together, pointing forward

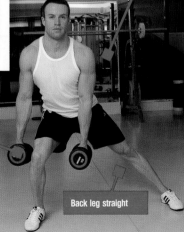

Body upright

Step to the side and bend your knee, keeping it in line with your foot

Back leg straight

LIGHT WEIGHTS

GO HEAVY

COMPOUND

ISOLATION

STABILISER

FORM ALERT

EXPLOSIVE

CORE

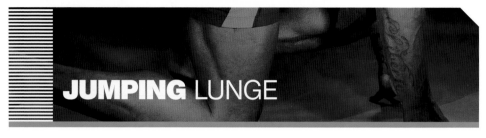

JUMPING LUNGE

86

Leaping from one lunge to another will build fast-twitch muscle fibres and also requires a lot of energy, so it's a great way of burning calories and improving cardiovascular fitness.

LIGHT WEIGHTS

GO HEAVY

COMPOUND

ISOLATION

STABILISER

FORM ALERT

EXPLOSIVE

CORE

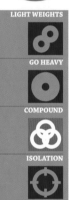

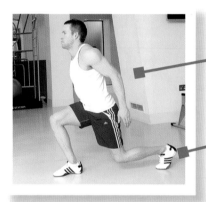

Start from a lunge position and draw your arms back, ready to jump

Feet pointing forwards

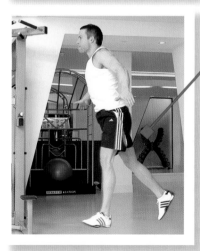

Jump up and swap leg postitions in mid-air

Land in a lunge on the opposite side and go straight into the next jump

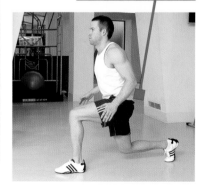

GYM BALL
BULGARIAN SPLIT SQUAT

87

Placing your back foot on a gym ball puts you in a very unstable position, so your muscles are required to work hard to keep you steady and maintain form.

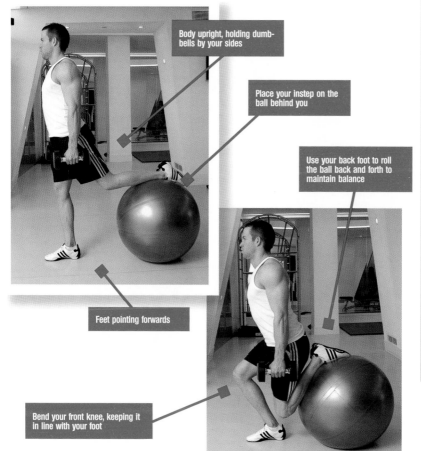

Body upright, holding dumbbells by your sides

Place your instep on the ball behind you

Use your back foot to roll the ball back and forth to maintain balance

Feet pointing forwards

Bend your front knee, keeping it in line with your foot

LIGHT WEIGHTS

GO HEAVY

COMPOUND

ISOLATION

STABILISER

FORM ALERT

EXPLOSIVE

CORE

ROMANIAN DEADLIFT

88

Target your hamstrings with a move that allows you to shift a lot of weight under control.

LIGHT WEIGHTS

GO HEAVY

COMPOUND

ISOLATION

STABILISER

FORM ALERT

EXPLOSIVE

CORE

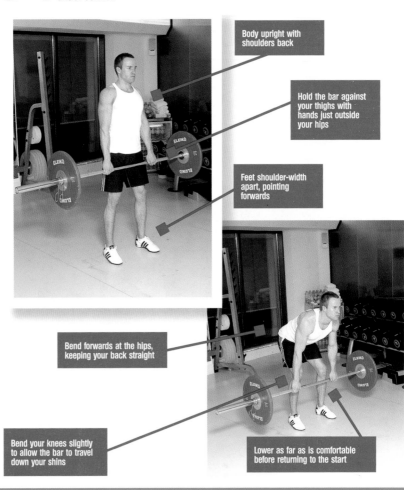

Body upright with shoulders back

Hold the bar against your thighs with hands just outside your hips

Feet shoulder-width apart, pointing forwards

Bend forwards at the hips, keeping your back straight

Bend your knees slightly to allow the bar to travel down your shins

Lower as far as is comfortable before returning to the start

GYM BALL
LEG CURL

89

Isolate your hamstrings with a move that looks simple but will soon exhaust your hams, especially if you do it immediately after Romanian deadlifts.

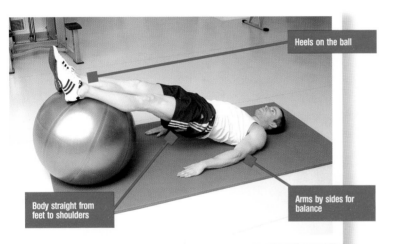

Heels on the ball

Body straight from feet to shoulders

Arms by sides for balance

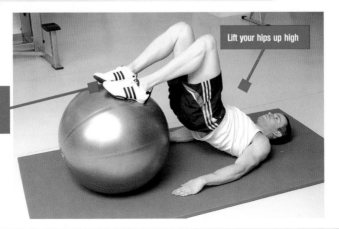

Lift your hips up high

Draw the ball into your backside using your heels

LIGHT WEIGHTS

GO HEAVY

COMPOUND

ISOLATION

STABILISER

FORM ALERT

EXPLOSIVE

CORE

101 BEST EXERCISES

ONE-LEG ROMANIAN DEADLIFT

90

Keep this move slow and controlled to build strength and stability in your glutes and hamstrings.

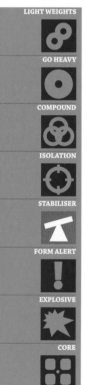
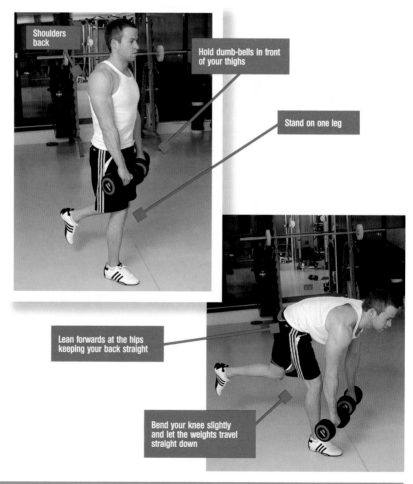

Shoulders back

Hold dumb-bells in front of your thighs

Stand on one leg

Lean forwards at the hips keeping your back straight

Bend your knee slightly and let the weights travel straight down

STANDING
CALF RAISE

91

Don't neglect your calves – add as much weight as you can manage to stimulate these hard-to-build muscles.

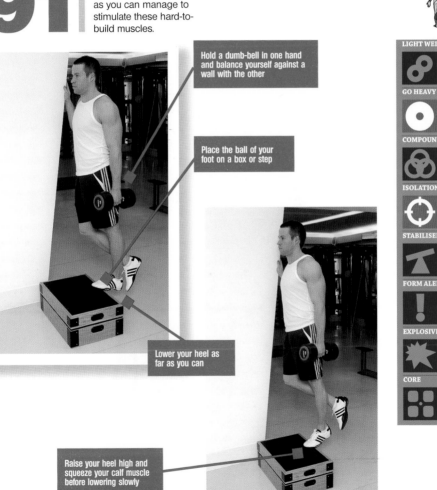

Hold a dumb-bell in one hand and balance yourself against a wall with the other

Place the ball of your foot on a box or step

Lower your heel as far as you can

Raise your heel high and squeeze your calf muscle before lowering slowly

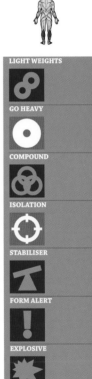

LIGHT WEIGHTS

GO HEAVY

COMPOUND

ISOLATION

STABILISER

FORM ALERT

EXPLOSIVE

CORE

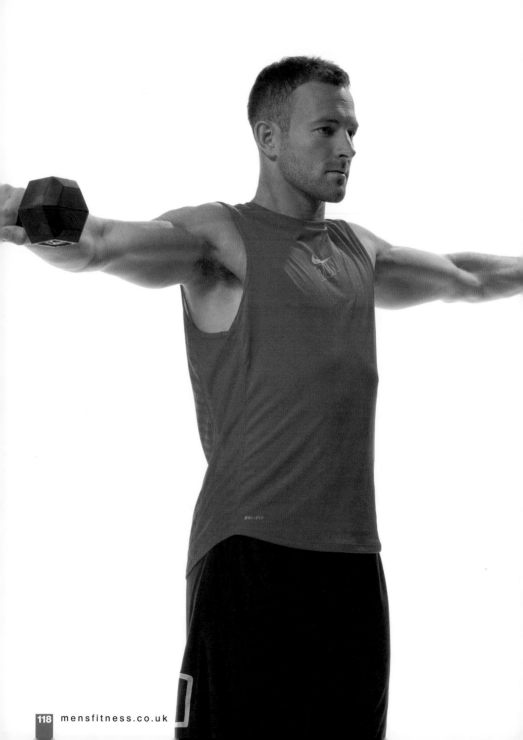

Shoulders

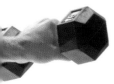

The main shoulder muscle, the deltoid, is a three-part muscle that goes around the shoulder joint. The anterior (front) deltoid starts on the collarbone, the medial (middle) deltoid starts on the top of the shoulder and the posterior (rear) deltoid starts on the shoulder blade.

The anterior deltoid is involved in pushing moves that also work the chest, such as the bench press. The medial deltoid is responsible lifting your arms straight overhead and the posterior deltoid is called upon when you raise your arms out from your sides.

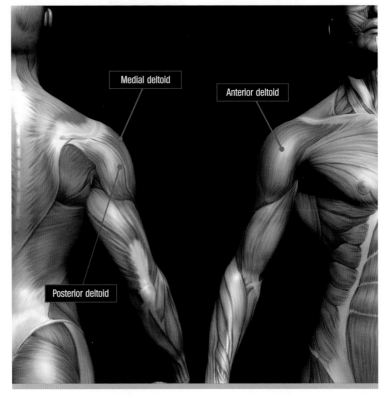

Medial deltoid

Anterior deltoid

Posterior deltoid

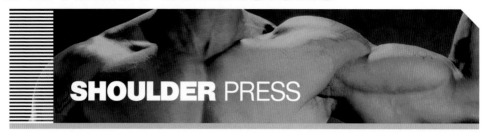

SHOULDER PRESS

92

This is the classic move for building bigger, stronger shoulders. Be sure to keep your core muscles contracted throughout to prevent excess stress on your lower back.

LIGHT WEIGHTS

GO HEAVY

COMPOUND

ISOLATION

STABILISER

FORM ALERT

EXPLOSIVE

CORE

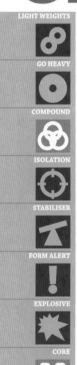

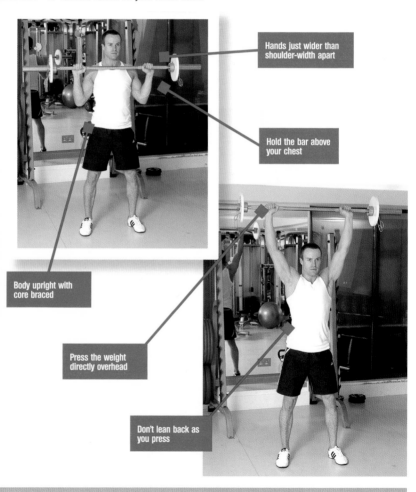

Hands just wider than shoulder-width apart

Hold the bar above your chest

Body upright with core braced

Press the weight directly overhead

Don't lean back as you press

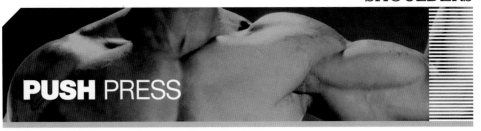

PUSH PRESS

93

Using your legs to initiate the move allows you press more weight, which in turn builds bigger muscles.

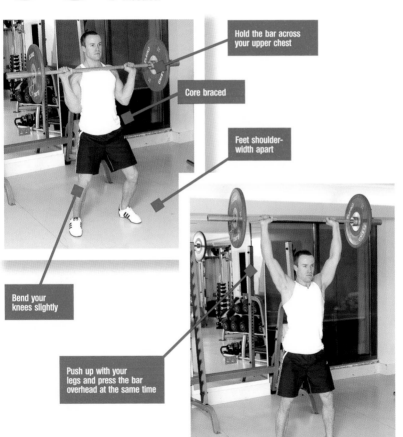

Hold the bar across your upper chest

Core braced

Feet shoulder-width apart

Bend your knees slightly

Push up with your legs and press the bar overhead at the same time

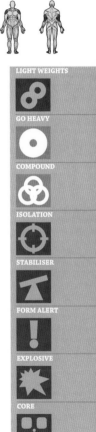

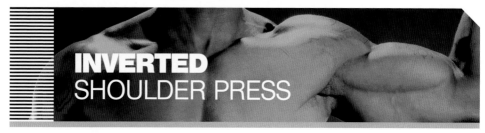

INVERTED
SHOULDER PRESS

94

When you don't have any weights to hand you can still build your shoulders. Just make sure you can control your own bodyweight so you don't fall on your face.

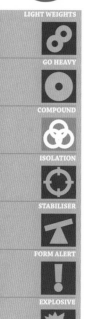

LIGHT WEIGHTS

GO HEAVY

COMPOUND

ISOLATION

STABILISER

FORM ALERT

EXPLOSIVE

CORE

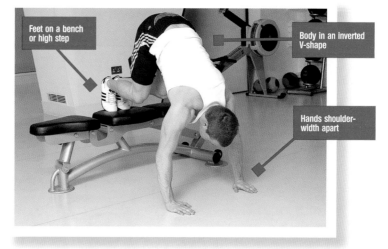

Feet on a bench or high step

Body in an inverted V-shape

Hands shoulder-width apart

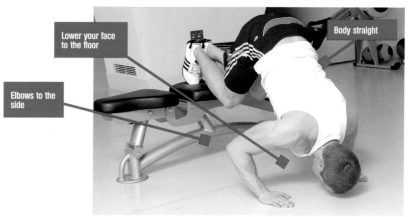

Lower your face to the floor

Body straight

Elbows to the side

SEATED DUMB-BELL
SHOULDER PRESS

95

The dumb-bells allow you to work each side of your shoulders independently, and also let your arms raise in their natural arc compared with using a barbell.

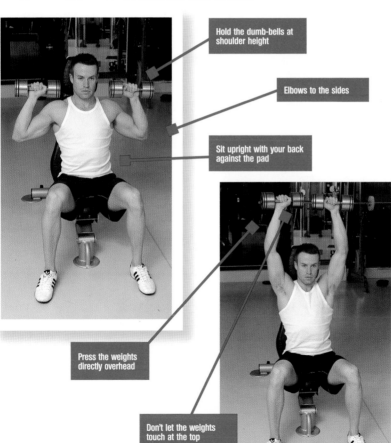

Hold the dumb-bells at shoulder height

Elbows to the sides

Sit upright with your back against the pad

Press the weights directly overhead

Don't let the weights touch at the top

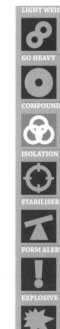

LIGHT WEIGHTS

GO HEAVY

COMPOUND

ISOLATION

STABILISER

FORM ALERT

EXPLOSIVE

CORE

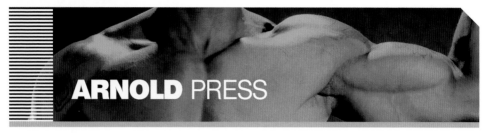

ARNOLD PRESS

96

This twist on the dumb-bell press combines a pushing motion with a rotational one, hitting your deltoids from several angles at once.

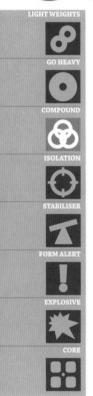

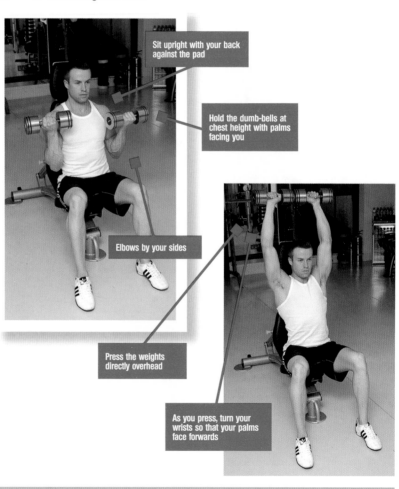

Sit upright with your back against the pad

Hold the dumb-bells at chest height with palms facing you

Elbows by your sides

Press the weights directly overhead

As you press, turn your wrists so that your palms face forwards

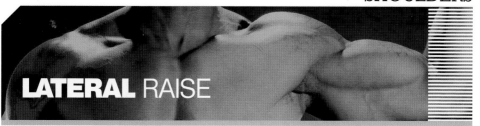

LATERAL RAISE

97

Isolate your deltoids with a single-joint move that gets harder the slower you do it.

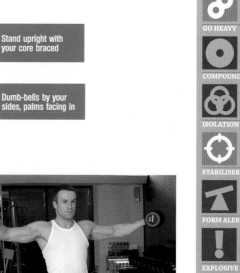

Stand upright with your core braced

Dumb-bells by your sides, palms facing in

Raise the weights directly to the sides to shoulder level

Keep a slight bend in your elbows as you lift

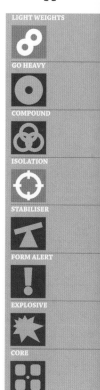

LIGHT WEIGHTS

GO HEAVY

COMPOUND

ISOLATION

STABILISER

FORM ALERT

EXPLOSIVE

CORE

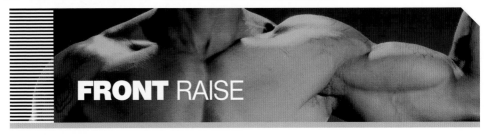

FRONT RAISE

98

Place the emphasis on your front deltoids, using light weights to protect the vulnerable rotator cuff muscles around your shoulder joint.

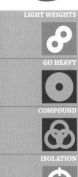

LIGHT WEIGHTS

GO HEAVY

COMPOUND

ISOLATION

STABILISER

FORM ALERT

EXPLOSIVE

CORE

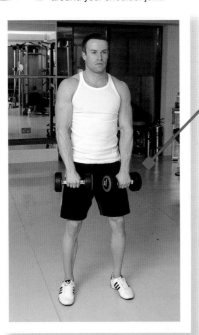

Hold dumb-bells in front of your thighs, palms facing you

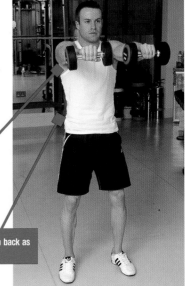

Raise the weights directly in front of you to shoulder height

Don't lean back as you lift

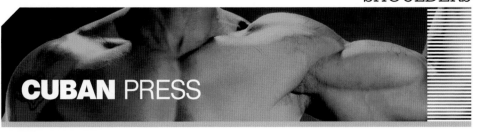

CUBAN PRESS

99

This complex move works your shoulder through several planes of motion, helping to strengthen your rotator cuffs – the muscles that stabilise your shoulder joint.

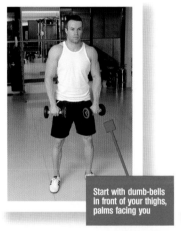

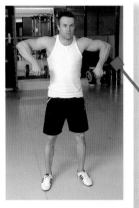

Raise your elbows to the sides, keeping your forearms pointing down

Start with dumb-bells in front of your thighs, palms facing you

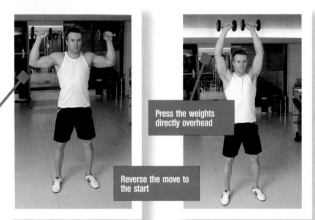

Rotate your upper arms until your forearms point up

Press the weights directly overhead

Reverse the move to the start

LIGHT WEIGHTS

GO HEAVY

COMPOUND

ISOLATION

STABILISER

FORM ALERT

EXPLOSIVE

CORE

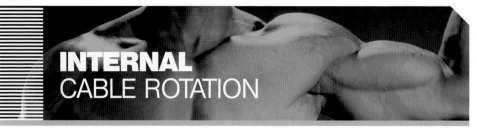

INTERNAL
CABLE ROTATION

100

Use this move as a warm-up for your shoulder joint before going on to do heavy lifts.

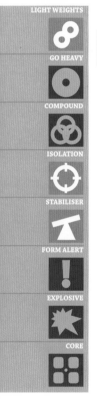

LIGHT WEIGHTS

GO HEAVY

COMPOUND

ISOLATION

STABILISER

FORM ALERT

EXPLOSIVE

CORE

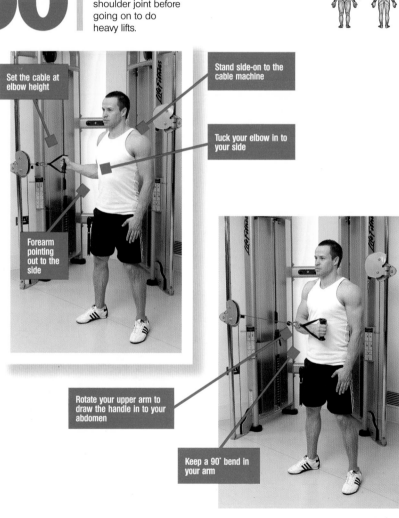

Set the cable at elbow height

Stand side-on to the cable machine

Tuck your elbow in to your side

Forearm pointing out to the side

Rotate your upper arm to draw the handle in to your abdomen

Keep a 90° bend in your arm

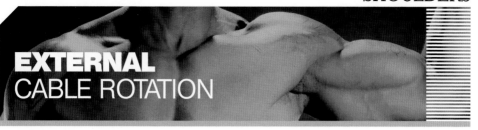

EXTERNAL
CABLE ROTATION

101

This works your rotator cuff muscles in the opposite plane to the internal rotation. Combine the two exercises together to give your shoulders a proper warm-up.

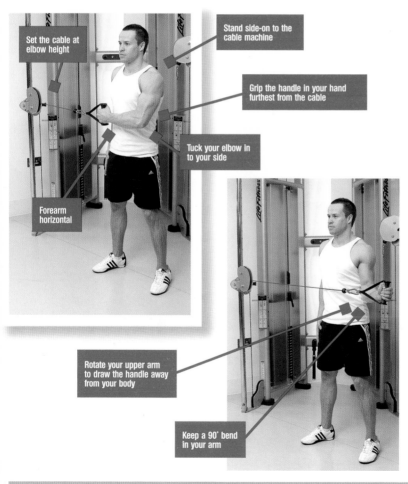

Set the cable at elbow height

Stand side-on to the cable machine

Grip the handle in your hand furthest from the cable

Tuck your elbow in to your side

Forearm horizontal

Rotate your upper arm to draw the handle away from your body

Keep a 90° bend in your arm

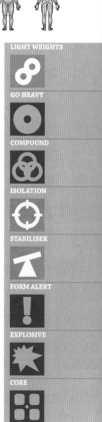

LIGHT WEIGHTS

GO HEAVY

COMPOUND

ISOLATION

STABILISER

FORM ALERT

EXPLOSIVE

CORE

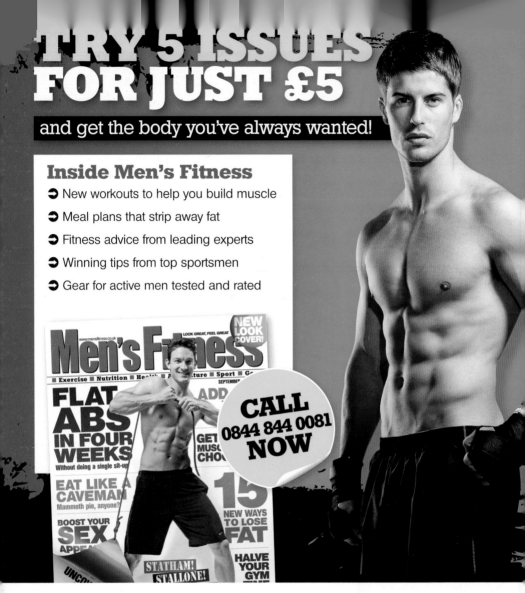

TRY 5 ISSUES FOR JUST £5

and get the body you've always wanted!

Inside Men's Fitness

- ➲ New workouts to help you build muscle
- ➲ Meal plans that strip away fat
- ➲ Fitness advice from leading experts
- ➲ Winning tips from top sportsmen
- ➲ Gear for active men tested and rated

CALL 0844 844 0081 NOW